W9-BAC-934

PHARMACOLOGY MADE INSANELY EASY

Loretta Manning
Sylvia Rayfield

Reviewed by
Nicole Blackwelder, PharmD.

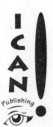
I CAN Publishing, Inc. • Bossier City, LA

I CAN Publishing, Inc.
P.O. Box 6192
Bossier City, LA 71171
866.428.5589

www.icanpublishing.com

Editorial Assistants: Teresa R. Davidson, Marcia Wright
Cartoon Illustrations: Eileen Burke, Pass Christian, MS; Teresa R. Davidson, Jamestown, NC
Cover Design: Teresa R. Davidson
Manuscript Preparation: Teresa R. Davidson
Production: Linda Seaman, Great Plains Book Manufacturing, Winfield, KS
Content Reviewer: Pattie Sue Carranza, RPh, CDE, Nicole Blackwelder, PharmD

©2005, by I CAN Publishing, Inc.
All rights reserved. No part of this book may be used or reproduced or transmitted in any form or by any means, electronic or mechanical, including photocopying, recording, or by an information storage and retrieval system without written permission from I CAN Publishing, Inc.

Printed in the United States of America
ISBN 0-9761029-0-0
Library of Congress Catalog Card Number: 2004116424

Pharmacology and Medicine are an ever-changing science. The authors and publisher have reviewed current and reliable sources and care has been taken to confirm the accuracy of the information presented and to describe generally accepted practices. The authors, editors, and publisher, however, disclaim all responsibility for errors, omissions, or consequences from application of the information in the book. *Pharmacology Made Insanely Easy* has been written to provide general principles of pharmacology and methods to remember this content. This book is not intended as a working guide for client drug administration. Many medications may be prescribed by health care providers for numerous and different indications beyond the scope of this book. Refer to the manufacturer's package insert for recommended drug dosage, route, total list of warnings and undesirable effects, and drug-drug interactions.

The butterfly on the cover signifies transformation. This book has been developed to assist the reader in transforming the study of pharmacology to an exciting and easy process.

ACKNOWLEDGMENTS

Janie Robinson, our Administrative Director and dear friend, who is always willing to step up to the plate to do whatever it takes to get a project done and make deadlines happen. Her love, support, and enthusiasm makes us smile daily.

Teresa Davidson, our Artist and dear friend, who painstakingly took all the words and scribbled ideas from my handwritten pad and entered them into the computer and developed the fun and memorable images. Teresa is always willing to go the extra mile to meet our deadlines.

Marcia Wright, our colleague and dear friend, for her support, sense of humor, inspiration, knowledge, and creativity.

Clara and John Fults who jump through hoops to get our books to the nurses, students, and faculty.

We want to thank our family, friends, nursing faculty, and students who have encouraged, supported, and inspired us during this project.

Loretta and Sylvia

I want to thank my dear husband, Randy, and my daughter, Erica, for their never-ending love and encouragement. Also to my beloved mother, Juanita Shera, who has always loved and supported me.

Loretta

Discovering new ways of learning and teaching pharmacology is a major reason for writing this book. We did not do this by ourselves. Some of these memory tools have been around for generations and we don't know their origins. We want to acknowledge and thank the colleagues, students, and friends who have contributed.

Pattie Akins, RN, MSN
Senior Lecturer
Baylor University, Louise Harrington School of Nursing
Dallas, TX

Julia Aucoin, DNS, RN, BC
Professional Development Consultant
Durham, NC

Marie Bremner, DSN, RN, CS
Professor of Nursing
Kennesaw State University, Kennesaw, GA

Karen Beard, MSN, RN, CS, GNP
Gerontological Nurse Practioner
Winston-Salem, NC

Candace J. Bishop, NP-C, RN, MS, CS
Well Star Health System
Marietta, GA

Marianne Call, RN, MN
Instructor
Charity School of Nursing/Delgado Community
    College, New Orleans, LA

Sharon Cooney, RN, ONC, MSN
Educational Consultant
Durham, NC

Diane DePew, DSN, RN
Director, Nursing Education Department
Holy Cross Hospital, Silver Springs, MD

Linda Fisher, MSN, RN
School Clinic Nurse
B. B. Harris Elementary, Duluth, GA

Darlene Franklin, MSN, RN
Assistant Professor of Nursing
Tennessee Technological University , Cookville, TN

Cecilia Hostetler, BA
Independent Contractor
Suwanee, GA

Joan Galbraith, MSN, RN, CS, GNP, ANP
Carol Woods Retirement Community,
Chapel Hill, NC
Ellen Lewis, MSN, RN, CS, GNP
Evercare, Atlanta, GA

Judy Mayo, RN, MSN
Assistant Professor
Sinclair College, Dayton, OH

Alita R. Maddox, APRN, MSN, PNP-C
Private Practice Nurse Practitioner
Bossier City, LA

Melora Mayo
Yale New Have Hospital
Children's Clinical Research Center

Kathy O'Leary Oller, RN, MSN
Nursing Instructor, Maternal Neo-Natal
    Nursing Coordinator
Florida Community College, Jacksonville, FL

Tina Rayfield, BS, PA-C
President, Sylvia Rayfield & Associates
Pensacola, FL

Vanice Roberts, DSN, RN
Assistant Dean
Kennesaw State University, Kennesaw, GA

John Shanley, MSN, RN, CS, GNP
Independent Consultant, Clinical Instructor
University of Memphis, Memphis, TN

Debra Shelton, MSN, RN, CNA, OCN-C, EdD(c)
Assistant Professor to RN and BSN Program
    Graduate Studies of Nursing
Northwestern State University, Shreveport, LA

Susan Snell, MSN, RN, BC, FNP
Assistant Professor
Northwestern State University, Shreveport, LA

Mayola L. Villarruel, RN, MSN, ANP
VA Chicago Health Care System
ABJOPC
Crown Point, IN

Marcia R. Wright, APRN, BC
Nursing Education Coordinator
Baptist Medical Center Beaches
Jacksonville Beach, FL

Dedicated with love to students, faculty, and health care professionals who are studying teaching or working with drug therapy.

When you are afraid of reviewing meds,
Read this book and soon you will lose your fear.
The right side of the page will soon get in your head
With the pertinent drug facts quickly becoming more clear.

I
CAN

Did is a word
  of achievement,
Won't is a word
  of retreat,
Might is a word
  of bereavement
Can't is a word
  of defeat,
Ought is a word
  of duty,
Try is a word
  each hour,
Will is a word
  of beauty,
Can is a word
  of power.

— Author Unknown

PREFACE
A Message to Our Readers

Pharmacology Made Insanely Easy , 2nd Edition has been written as a result of numerous requests from students, graduates, and faculty who have struggled to learn or teach pharmacology. As we work with groups across the country, the common concern is "there is just too much to remember about all the drugs". While using our teaching strategies during our pharmacology courses, we are told routinely that learners can remember more pharmacology after a few hours with us than they could at the end of a semester of a pharmacology course. Learners report spending hours trying to memorize subtle differences between drugs with similar actions, undesirable effects, etc. We have designed this book, utilizing our strategies, to make life easier for any learner or professional teaching their clients how to safely manage these medications or teaching students pharmacology.

Our experience with thousands of learners each year has helped us develop images and strategies that accelerate the learning process. The format is insanely easy! On the left page is the "bottom line information" about the medications. The image or memory tool is on the right page. Our intent for this book is not for it to be a drug book or pharmacology textbook. This book has been designed to help **simplify** volumes of information as well as to assist you in organizing some of the most pertinent information. In order to assist you in keeping focused on your goal, we have not included exhaustive lists of undesirable effects, doses, routes, or long lists of drug incompatibilities.

We have had a lot of fun working on this project. We look forward to hearing from you. Our web site is www.ican publishing.com. We would love to hear from you regarding recommendations for future editions.

Loretta Manning
Sylvia Rayfield

"THE IMPORTANT THING IN SCIENCE IS NOT SO MUCH TO OBTAIN NEW FACTS AS TO DISCOVER NEW WAYS OF THINKING ABOUT THEM."

Sir William Bragg

TABLE OF CONTENTS

HINTS ON HOW TO USE
PHARMACOLOGY MADE INSANELY EASY

As we prepared this book, our ultimate goal was to make learning pharmacology fun and easy! As we waded through volumes of research and information on pharmacology, we realized there were some similarities that were applicable to all medications. Rather than repeating these facts with each category and/or medication, we are using the mnemonic "COMPLIANCE". This will assist you in remembering the facts that must be considered for each category of medicines.

When you are reviewing pharmacology, do you ever feel like you are having a "power outage" in your brain? To simplify the content, in several sections of this book we have developed a concept page. This information is pertinent to all of the medications in that category. The left side of the page will review the mnemonic in more detail. This information will not be repeated throughout every category in order to simplify the content. The mnemonic, however, will be referred to in the text of the drug on the left page. The categories that will have these concept pages include: antibiotics, anticoagulants, antidiabetic agents, antidepressants, antihypertensives, bronchodilators, agents used for chemotherapy, and diuretics.

As we work with graduates across the United States in our review courses, a common request is to have a list outlining the drugs that can cause damage to specific body organs. This has been developed and provided for you in this book. It includes specific drugs that can cause hepatotoxicity, nephrotoxicity, and ototoxicity. Common drug-drug and food-drug interactions are also included. There will be an image of a sun for drugs that may have an undesirable effect of photosensitivity. The Joint Commission on Accreditation of Healthcare Organizations recently released a list of medications with the highest risk of injury when misused. These high-alert medications were divided into six groups: insulins, opiates, antineoplastics, injectable potassium chloride or phosphate, intravenous anticoagulants, and sodium chloride solutions stronger than 0.9%. These categories were established from a study performed by the Institute for Safe Medication Practices. To assist the reader in identifying these drugs, each drug or category will have an image of the yield sign at the top of the page with the words "HIGH ALERT".

We hope you enjoy this book, and it helps you to study and remember facts about pharmacology. Please feel free to notify us if you have additional requests or recommendations for our future publications. We would love to hear from you.

Learning pharmacology in our book is very fun;
Just look for specific images such as the sun.
The images will help you recall important facts,
And prevent you from having to read a very large text.

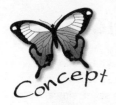

Concept

C hildren—safety

O bserve, report, teach about undesirable effects

M eds—no over-the-counter w/o consultation

P regnancy/lactating are out with meds

L iver must be intact

I nteractions—pharmacological, assess and teach

A llergies—assess; do not administer med if allergic

N utrition must be considered; no crushing sustained release tablets

C ompliance with time and taking full course

E lderly—safety, evaluate outcomes for all meds

©2001 I CAN Publishing, Inc.

"DO NOT USE" ABBREVIATIONS

Following is a list of frequently used abbreviations that should not be used by institutions as they can be easily misinterpreted:

Abbreviations	Preferred Term
μ (for microgram)	Write **mcg**
T.I.W. for three times weekly	Write **3** (or Three) **Times Weekly**
Trailing zero	Do not use zeros after decimal point (for example, X instead of X.0)
cc for cubic centimeter	Write **ml** for milliliters
IU for International Unit	Write the word **International Unit**
U for Unit	Write the word **Unit**

Abbreviations	Preferred Term
QD for Every Day	Write **Every Day** or **Daily**
Q.O.D. for Every Other Day	Write **Every Other Day**
Leading zero	Use zeros before the decimal point (for example, 0.X instead of .X)
MS & MS04 for morphine	Write **morphine sulfate**
MGS04	Write **Magnesium Sulfate**

The Institute for Safe Medication Practices (ISMP) has published a list of dangerous abbreviations relating to medication use that it recommends should be explicitly prohibited. This list is available on the ISMP website: **http://www.ismp.org**.

Source: Nicole Blackwelder, PharmD, Baptist Medical Center, Beaches, Jacksonville, FL. Reprinted with permission. Adapted from the Joint Commission on Accrediation of Healthcare Organizations "Do Not Use" Abbreviations, www.jcho.org.

PHARMACOKINETICS

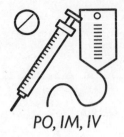

PO, IM, IV

Pharmacology Made Insanely Easy will not review routes or dosages. This information can be found in drug books or pharmacology references.

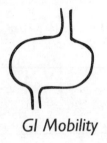

GI Mobility

Alterations in the gastric motility may have effects on how the drugs are absorbed.

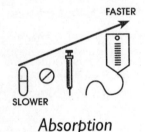

Absorption

Absorption can also be affected by route of administration or an impairment in circulation.

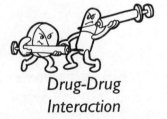

Drug-Drug Interaction

Gut=pH of stomach 4–5. Some drugs require an acidic enviroment for absorption (i.e., tetracycline), raising the pH will alter the absorption.

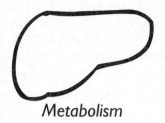

Metabolism

Many drugs pass initially through the liver prior to being available to tissue. Liver disease may ↑ or ↓ action of a drug depending on the metabolism in the body. Infants and elderly have ↓ liver function.

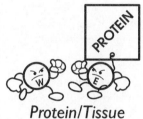
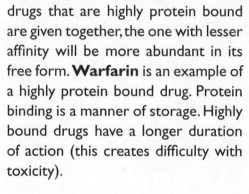

Protein/Tissue Binding

Many drugs bind to protein. When 2 drugs that are highly protein bound are given together, the one with lesser affinity will be more abundant in its free form. **Warfarin** is an example of a highly protein bound drug. Protein binding is a manner of storage. Highly bound drugs have a longer duration of action (this creates difficulty with toxicity).

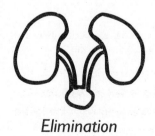

Elimination

Routes of elimination include the kidney, lungs, skin, GI tract, breast milk. Kidney is the major route of excretion. Adequate blood flow to the kidney and renal function are major contributors to drug clearance. If the drug is excreted unchanged such as digoxin or potassium, the renal function must be intact. Elderly have ↓ renal function.

DRUG-DRUG INTERACTIONS

The complexity of modern pharmacology is a growing concern as the list of drug-drug interactions and food-drug interactions continue to grow. **"The Mad War"** on the next page outlines some of the drugs commmonly involved in drug-drug interactions. There are several factors influencing the drug interactions including the absorption of the intestine, competition for plasma protein binding, drug metabolism, action at the receptor site, renal elimination, and electrolyte imbalance.

Absorption of the intestine: Antacids or foods containing aluminum, calcium, or magnesium may bind with tetracycline, decreasing the absorption of the antibiotic. Some drugs require an acidic environment for absorption; increasing the pH will alter the absorption. (pH of stomach is 4–5).

Competition for plasma protein binding: One of the major reasons for drug-drug interactions is the binding of many drugs to proteins, mainly albumin proteins. When 2 drugs that are highly protein bound are administered together, the one with a lesser affinity will be more abundant in its free form. As an individual ages, the number of binding sites on blood proteins is finite. An example of a highly protein bound medication is warfarin.

Drug metabolism: The monoamine oxidase inhibitors prevent the biotransformation of tyramine. Tyramine is present in products such as over-the-counter cold medicines, aged cheese, liver, preserved meats (i.e., bologna, pepperoni, sausage), red wine, tea, colas containing caffeine, chocolate drinks, avocado, figs, pear extracts, etc. This lack of biotransformation of tyramine may result in a hypertensive crisis.

Action at the receptor site: There are many drugs that will intensify or antagonize the action of another drug. For example, alcohol will increase the effects of CNS depressants; antihistamines will decrease the effects of histamine.

Renal elimination: An example of a drug altering renal excretion is probenecid (Benemid) which inhibits the renal clearance of penicillin.

Electrolyte imbalance: Potassium sparing diuretics in combination with ace inhibitors may result in hyperkalemia. An alteration in the sodium level will alter the range of lithium. The use of loop diuretics may result in hypokalemia, which predisposes the client to the potential risk for digitalis toxicity.

DRUG-DRUG INTERACTIONS

T ricyclic antidepressants

H $_2$ Histamine Antagonist
(Tagamet)

E thanol
rythromycin

M A O inhibitors

A minophylline
spirin

D igoxin
ilantin
iuretics

W arfarin

A zole (antifungal)
ntacids

R ifampin

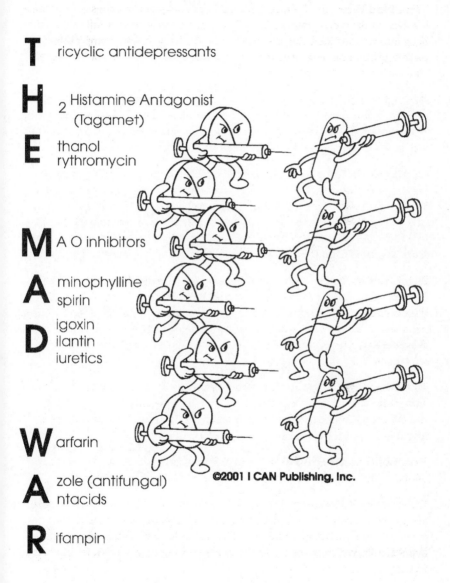

©2001 I CAN Publishing, Inc.

FOOD-DRUG INTERACTIONS

Drug	Foods to Avoid

Antacids
calcium carbonate
(Tums used as calcium
supplement)

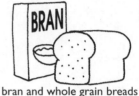

bran and whole grain breads

Antibiotics
erythromycin, penicillin

citrus fruit, colas and any food

Tetracycline

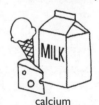

calcium

Anticoagulants
warfarin (coumadin)

vitamin K

MAO Inhibitors

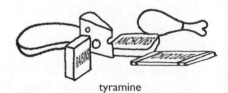

tyramine

DRUGS THAT CAN CAUSE NEPHROTOXICITY

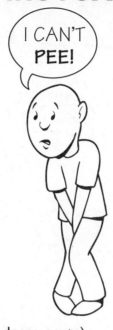

acetaminophen (high doses, acute)

acyclovir, parenteral (Zovirax)

aminoglycocides

amphotericin B, parenteral (Fungizone)

analgesic combinations containing acetaminophen, aspirin or
   other salicylates in high doses, chronically

ciprofloxacin

cisplatin (Platinol)

methotrexate (high doses)

nonsteroidal anti-inflammatory drugs (NSAIDs)

rifampin

sulfonamides

tetracyclines (exceptions are doxycycline and minocycline)

vancomycin, parenteral (Vancocin)

DRUGS THAT CAN CAUSE HEPATOTOXICITY

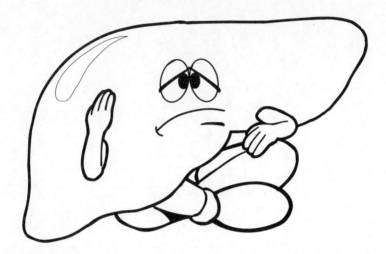

ACE inhibitors
acetaminophen
alcohol
iron overdose
erythromycins
estrogens
fluconazole (Diflucan)
isoniazid (INH)
itraconazole (Sporanox)
ketoconazole (Nizoral)
nonsteroidal anti-inflammatory drugs (NSAIDs)
phenothiazines
phenytoin (Dilantin)
rifampin (Rifadin)
sulfamethooxazole and trimethoprin (Bactrin, Septra)
sulfonamides

DRUGS THAT CAN CAUSE OTOTOXICITY

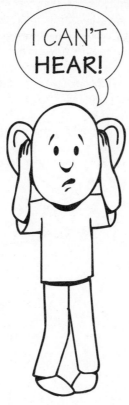

aminoglycosides
bumetanide, parenteral (Bumex)
cisplatin
erythromycin (renal impairment and high doses)
ethacrynic acid (Edecrin)
furosemide (Lasix)
hydroxychloroquine (Plaquenil)
nonsteroidal anti-inflammatory drugs (NSAIDs)
salicylates (chronic high doses, overuse)
vancomycin, parenteral (high doses and renal impairment)

POLYPHARMACY

Polypharmacy is the prescription of numerous medications. Numerous medications may be necessary when a client has several medical disorders, when various medications improve the symptoms of a specific disease, or when one medication improves the action of another. Multiple medication regimens, however, frequently lack rationale for each medication. Elderly clients typically have more than one provider of health care, which may result in poorly coordinated care. The major problem is that medicines administered to relieve nonspecific symptomatology or the undesirable effects of other medicines are believed to be major contributing factors to undesirable effects resulting from polypharmacy.

As you review pharmacology, polypharmacy and drug-drug interactions must always be part of the assessment and planning. While polypharmacy will not be repeated with the categories and individual medication reviews, it is a major part of the management.

POLLY PHARMACY

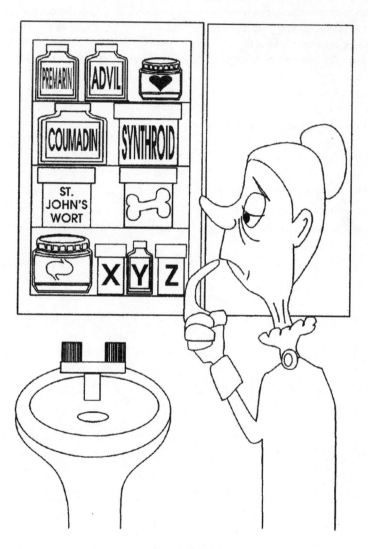

©2001 I CAN Publishing, Inc.

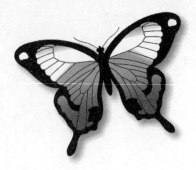

Do the one thing you think you cannot do. Fail at it. Try again. Do better the second time. The only people who never tumble are those who never mount the high wire.

Oprah Winfrey

Cardiovascular Agents

CHF DRUGS

Action: Inhibits the sodium-potassium ATPase, resulting in an increase in cardiac contraction. Decreases heart rate.

Indication: CHF, atrial fibrillation and/or flutter, and paroxysmal atrial contractions.

Warnings: Ventricular fibrillation/tachycardia; severe bradycardia; digitalis toxicity; caution with impaired renal or hepatic function; incomplete AV block; elderly; or electrolyte abnormality ($\downarrow$ K$^+$, $\downarrow$ Mg^{++}, $\uparrow$ Ca^{++}), or acute MI.

Undesirable Effects: Anorexia, nausea (first signs of adult toxicity), upset stomach (first sign of toxicity in older child). Vertigo, headache, depression, muscle weakness, drowsiness, confusion (may be first sign in the elderly client). Bradycardia, ECG changes, heart block. Photophobia, yellow-green halos around visual images, flashes of light.

Other Significant Information: $\downarrow$ K$^+$, $\downarrow$ Mg^{++}, and $\uparrow$ Ca^{++} may be associated with digitalis toxicity. Administer separately from antacids (1 to 2 hours apart). Use cautiously with calcium channel blockers or beta blockers. Numerous drug interactions may occur. (*Refer to a Drug Handbook for the specifics. This is beyond the scope of this book.*) Incompatible with dobutamine.

Interventions: Monitor K+, Mg++, ECG, liver/renal function tests, drug level (therapeutic level 0.5–2.0 ng/ml, toxicity is > 2.0 ng/mL). Before each dose, assess apical pulse for full minute; record and report changes in rate or rhythm. Withhold drug and contact provider if pulse is < 60/minute (adults) or <90/minute (children) (unless provider has outlined specific parameters). Weigh daily, monitor I & O, and signs of CHF. Antidote: use digoxin immune FAB (Digibind or Digifab) for life-threatening digoxin intoxication (> 10 mg/ml or K$^+$ 7.5 mg/L).

Education: Avoid giving with meals. Teach to take pulse correctly and report if pulse is out of parameter. Weigh every other day and record. Restrict alcohol, sodium, smoking. Consult with provider prior to taking OTC meds. Eat foods rich in potassium. Wear medical alert tag. Emphasize importance of regular checkups. Report N & V or "yellow" vision.

Evaluation: A normal sinus rhythm on ECG. Clinical improvement as evidenced by no S3, edema, etc. Cardiomegaly decreased.

Drugs: digitoxin (Crystodigin); digoxin (Lanoxin)

LIZZY DIGGY

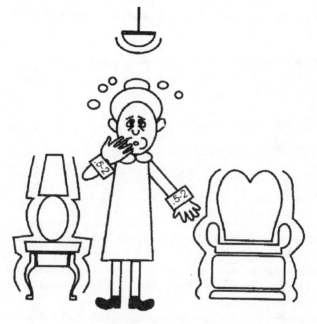

©2001 I CAN Publishing, Inc.

D ig level 2 ng/ml or greater is toxic

I ncreases myocardial contractility

G I or CNS signs indicate adverse effects

Lizzy Diggy is a little old lady that does not do well on DIG. She gets confused, dizzy, nauseated and sees halos and different colored lights.

NATRECOR

Action: Uses DNA technology; human B-type natriuretic peptide binds to the receptor in the vascular smooth muscle and endothelial cells, leading to smooth muscle relaxation.

Indications: Acutely decompensated CHF.

Warnings: Hypersensitivity, cardiogenic shock or BP<90 mm Hg as primary therapy.

Undesirable Effects: Headache, insomnia, hypotension, tachycardia, dysrhythmias, ventricular tachycardia, nausea, vomiting, rash, sweating, pruritus. Increased cough, hemoptysis, apnea.

Other Specific Information: Increased symptomatic hypotension with ACE inhibitors.

Interventions: Assess PCWP, RAP, cardiac index, MPAP, BP, heart rate during treatment until stable. Do not administer nesiritide through a central heparin coated cath. Infuse heparin through a separate line. Prime IV fluid with infusion of 25 ml before connecting to client's vascular accesss port and before bolus dose or IV infusion. Use within 24 hours of reconstitution.

Education: Educate client regarding the purpose of the medication and the expected results.

Evaluation: Client will expect an improvement in the CHF with an improvement in the PCWP, RAP, and MPAP.

Drug: nesiritide (Natrecor)

NATRECOR

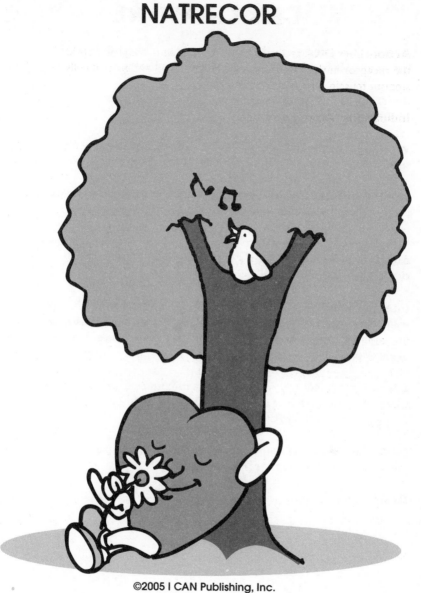

©2005 I CAN Publishing, Inc.

As you can see, the heart is relaxing and enjoying nature as a result of natrecor. Natrecor is effective in treating decompensated heart failure.

DOBUTAMINE

Action: Stimulates beta$_1$ adrenergic receptors (myocardial) to increase contractility but with relatively minor effect on heart rate.

Indications: Short-term management of heart failure due to decreased contractility.

Warnings: Hypersensitivity to bisulfites; idiopathic hypertrophic subaortic stenosis; myocardial infarction; atrial fibrillation; pregnancy; lactation; children.

Undesirable effects: ↑ BP, dysrhythmias, tachycardia, headache, angina pectoris, dyspnea, nausea, vomiting.

Other specific information: Beta-adrenergic inhibitors will negate the effects; nitroprusside use has a synergic effect; ↑ risk of dysrhythmias with cyclopropane, halothane, MAO inhibitors, oxytocics, or tricyclic antidepressants.

Interventions: Monitor pulse, blood pressure, respirations, ECG pattern, pulmonary capillary wedge pressure, central venous pressure, cardiac output, urine output, peripheral pulses, and color and temperature of extremities; monitor potassium, electrolytes, BUN, creatinine, and prothrombin time.

Education: Immediately report signs and symptoms of impending myocardial infarction or of worsening of heart failure; notify healthcare provider of pain or discomfort in the site of administration.

Evaluation: ↑ cardiac output; improved hemodynamic parameters; ↑ urine output; improvement in heart failure.

Drugs: Dobutrex

DOBUTAMINE

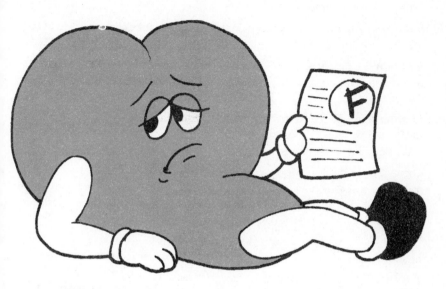

F ailure (heart)

A ngina, arrhythmia—undesirable effect

I ncreases contractility, blood pressure

L ook for an increase in cardiac and urine output

DOPAMINE

Action: Adrenergic. Causes increased cardiac output. Acts on beta 1 and alpha receptors. This results in vasoconstriction in blood vessels; low dose causes renal and mesenteric vasodiation; beta 1 stimulates the production of an inotropic effect with an increased cardiac output.

Indication: Shock; increased perfusion; hypotension. Unlabeled use: COPD, RDS in infants.

Warnings: **HIGH ALERT DRUG** Hypersensitivity. Ventricular fibrillation, tachydysrhythmias, pheochromocytoma. Arterial embolism, peripheral vascular disease.

Undesirable Effects: Headache, Palpitations, tachycardia, hypertension, angina, wide QRS complex, peripheral vasoconstriction. Nausea and vomiting, diarrhea. Necrosis, tissue sloughing with extravasation, gangrene with prolonged use, dyspnea.

Other Specific Information: Do not use within 2 wks of MAOIs, phenytoin; hypertensive crisis may result. Dysrhythmias: general anesthetics. Severe hypertension with ergots. Decreased action of dopamine with beta blockers and alpha blockers. Increased blood pressure with oxytocics. Increased pressor effect with tricyclics, MAOIs.

Interventions: Assess for hypovolemia; if this is a problem correct first. Assess oxygenation and perfusion deficit (check blood pressure, chest pain, dizziness, loss of consciousness). Assess heart failure: S3 gallop, dyspnea, neck vein distention, bibasilar crackles in clients with CHF, cardiomyopathy. I & O, if urine output decreases, without decrease in blood pressure, drug may need to be reduced. ECG during administration continuously; if blood pressure increases, drug should be decreased. B/P and pulse q 5 min after parenteral route. CVP and PWP during infusion if possible. Paresthesias and coldness of extremities; peripheral blood flow may decrease. Injection site: if tissue sloughs administer phentolamine mixed with NS. If overdose occurs, discontinue IV and give a short acting alpha adrenergic blocker.

Education: Instruct the family and client the reason for drug administration.

Staff Education: Do not confuse dopamine with dobutamine. Dopamine is a unique drug and different from the other adrenergic agonists because its actions depends on the dose. Doses of 5 to 10 micorgrams per kg per min. stimulate alpha receptors. Doses of 2–3 micorgrams per kg per min. stimulate dopaminergic receptors, causing dilation of the mesenteric and renal arteries. Dopamine is frequently used to increase blood flow to the kidneys when renal insufficiency is present or to prevent renal failure from shock.

Evaluation: Increased B/P with stabilization; increased urine output.

Drug: dopamine (Dopamine HCl, Intropin)

DO**PAM**INE

D ilation of pupils

R ate of heart will increase

A rterioles constrict (↑ BP)

G I tract motility

Help! I'm in shock!

PAM

MR. ARTERY

©2005 I CAN Publishing, Inc.

" Fight or Flight" angel, PAM, is throwing a life raft to the artery, constricting the artery because it was in shock and over dilated. She will "DRAG" the artery to shore. "DRAG" will assist you in remembering the responses of the alpha and B 1 receptor effects.

EPINEPHRINE

Action: Stimulates alpha- and beta-adrenergic receptors to (1) cause bronchodilation and vasoconstriction, (2) maintain pulse and blood pressure, (3) localize and prolong local and spinal anesthetic, and (4) reverse hypersensitivity reaction.

Indications: Asthma and COPD (maintenance of airway); allergic reactions; cardiac arrest; adjunct to local or spinal anesthesia; antiglaucoma.

Warnings: Use with caution in cardiac disease, hypertension, hyperthyroidism, and diabetes mellitus. Elderly persons may require ↓ dosage. Concurrent use with other adrenergic medications will have a synergistic effect. Beta-adrenergic inhibitors may negate the effect of epinephrine. Concurrent use with MAO inhibitors may cause a hypertensive crisis.

Undesirable effects: Nervousness, restlessness, tremors, angina, dysrhythmias, hypertension, tachycardia, headache, insomnia, paradoxical bronchospasm, nausea, vomiting, and hyperglycemia.

Other specific information: Check dosage, concentration, and route of administration carefully prior to administration. During treatment for anaphylactic shock, volume replacement should occur concurrently with epinephrine administration.

Interventions: Monitor pulmonary status before, during, and after bronchodilation treatment; monitor hemodynamic status during and after use for treatment of shock, hypotension, and/or cardiac arrest; treatment may cause ↓ K, ↑ glucose, and ↑ lactic acid.

Education: Take as directed; notify healthcare provider if symptoms are not relieved; discuss with healthcare provider before taking any over-the-counter medication.

Evaluation: Relief or prevention of bronchospasm; easier breathing; prevention of or ↓ frequency of acute asthma attacks; reversal of signs and symptoms of anaphylaxis; ↑ cardiac output and rate in cardiac resuscitation.

Drugs: Adrenalin, Ana-Gard, AsthmaHaler Mist, AsthmaNefrin, Bronitin Mist, Bronkaid Mist, Epifrin, Epinal, EpiPen, Eppy/N, Glaucon, microNefrin, Nephron, Primatene, Racepinephine, S-2, Sus-Phrine, Vaponefrin.

EPINEPHRINE

N ervousness—undesirable effect

A ngina, arrhythmia—undesirable effect

S ugar↑

C ardiac arrest

A llergic reaction

R espiratory—bronchodialator

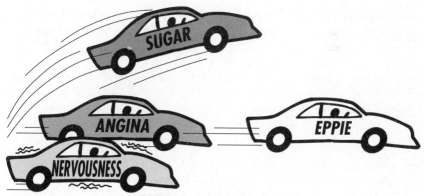

©2005 I CAN Publishing, Inc.

Three of these "NASCARS" experienced collisions (undesirable effects) from epinephrine. Eppie was able to finish the race and achieve desirable outcomes without any collisions (undesirable effects).

NOREPINEPHRINE

Action: Vasopressor; stimulates alpha- and beta-adrenergic receptors to cause vasoconstriction maintaining blood pressure.

Indications: Management of shock.

Warnings: Use with MAO inhibitors may result in hypertension; beta-adrenergic blockers may inhibit therapeutic effects; use cautiously in patients with underlying cardiovascular disease, uncorrected dysrhythmias, or hypovolemia due to fluid deficit.

Undesirable effects: Angina, hypertension, tachycardia, dysrhythmias; extravasation may cause severe irritation, necrosis, and sloughing of tissue.

Other specific information: If extravasation occurs, infiltrate area with 10–15 ml of 0.9% NaCl with 5–10 mg of phentolamine.

Interventions: Monitor blood pressure, heart rate, respirations, ECG, and hemodynamic parameters every 5–15 minutes; monitor urine output hourly; administer into a large vein to decrease risk of extravasation; correct hypovolemia before administering drug; administer via infusion pump to ensure precise dosing; titrate to patient response (blood pressure, heart rate, urine output, peripheral perfusion, cardiac output, and presence of ectopic activity).

Education: Immediately report signs and symptoms of chest pain or dyspnea; notify healthcare provider of pain or discomfort in the site of administration.

Evaluation: ↑ blood pressure, ↑ in peripheral circulation, ↑ in urine output.

Drugs: Levophed, Levarternol

NOREPINEPHRINE

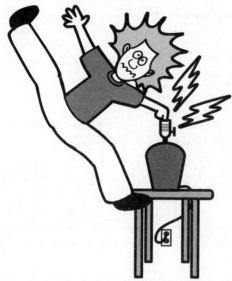

S timulates alpha and beta adrenergic receptors

H ypovolemia—should be corrected before using drug

O utput of urine & cardiac should ↑

C onstriction of blood vessels

K orrect dysrhythmias before using

NITROGLYCERIN

Action: Relaxes the vascular smooth system. ↓ myocardial demand for oxygen. ↓ left ventricular preload by dilating veins, thus indirectly ↓ afterload.

Indications: Angina pectoris.

Warnings: Hypersensitivity. Closed-angle glaucoma, severe anemia, hypotension, early MI, head trauma, ICP, pregnancy, renal or hepatic disease.

Undesirable Effects: Headache (most common), hypotension, postural hypotension, syncope, dizziness, weakness, reflex tachycardia, paradoxical bradycardia. Sublingual: burning, tingling sensation in mouth. Ointment: erythematous, vesicular and pruritic lesions.

Other Specific Information: ↑ effect with alcohol, antihypertensive agents, beta blockers, calcium blockers. ↓ effect of heparin.

Interventions: Record characteristics and precipitating factors of anginal pain. Monitor BP and apical pulse before administration and periodically after dose. Have client sit or lie down if taking drug for the first time. Client must have continuing EKG monitoring for IV administration. Cardioverter / defibrillator must not be discharged through paddle electrode overlying Nitro-Bid ointment or the Transderm-Nitro patch (may cause burns on client). Assist with ambulating if dizzy.

Education: Avoid alcohol. Teach to recognize symptoms of hypotension. Advise to make position changes slowly and to avoid prolonged standing. Teach about the form of nitroglycerin prescribed. Oral: Instruct to take on an empty stomach with a full glass of water. Do not chew tablet. Sublingual: Instruct to take at first sign of anginal pain. May be repeated every 5 minutes to a maximum of 3 doses. If the client doesn't experience relief, advise to seek medical assistance immediately. A stinging or biting sensation may indicate the tablet is fresh. With newer SL nitroglycerin, the biting sensation may not be present. Protect drug from light, moisture, and heat. Instruct to apply Transderm-Nitro patch once a day, usually in the AM. Rotation of sites is necessary. (*Refer to Drug Handbook for detail steps with all forms.*)

Evaluation: The client will report a decrease in frequency and severity of anginal attacks along with an increase in activity tolerance.

Drugs: nitroglycerin **intravenous** (Nitro-Bid IV, Tridil); **sublingual** (Nitrostat); **sustained-release** (Nitroglyn, Nitrong, Nitro-Time); **topical** (Nitro-Bid, Nitrol, Nitrong, Nitrostat); **transdermal** (Deponit, Minitran, Nitro-Dur, Nitrodisc, Transderm-Nitro, Nitro-Derm); **translingual** (Nitrolingual); **transmucosal** (Nitrogard)

ANDY ANGINA

ACTION

Relaxes vascular smooth muscle

↓ venous return

↓ arterial BP

↓ left ventricular workload

↓ myocardial oxygen consumption

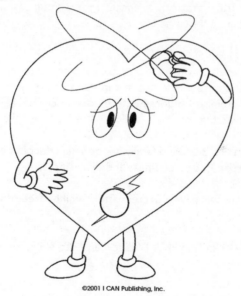

©2001 I CAN Publishing, Inc.

Nitroglycerin is given to decrease Andy's angina. Andy is experiencing some of the undesirable effects from nitroglycerin: headache, syncope, weakness, nausea, and hypotension.

ANTIARRHYTHMIC: LIDOCAINE

Action: Decreases cardiac excitability, cardiac conduction is delayed in the ventricle. Decreases automaticity of ventricular cells.

Indications: Ventricular dysrhythmias such as PVCs, ventricular tachycardia, and ventricular fibrillation.

Warnings: Advanced atrioventricular blocks, CHF, hepatic disorder, elderly client.

Undesirable Effects: Bradycardia, tachycardia, hypotension, confusion, drowsiness (*1st sign of toxicity*), dizziness, nausea, vomiting, seizures (*severe toxicity*), cardiac arrest.

Other Specific Information: ↑ effects with ranitidine, cimetidine. ↑ risk of toxicity with beta-adrenergic blockers, (LOL's).

Interventions: Monitor EKG, BP, pulse, and rhythm continuously. Monitor serum lidocaine levels throughout therapy; therapeutic range 1.5–5 mcg/mL. Monitor intake and output. Do not mix in same syringe with amphotericin B or cefazolin. Administer Lidocaine IV. In case of circulatory depression, have dopamine available.

Education: Instruct client and family about drug. Recommend client walk with another person due to dizziness and drowsiness.

Evaluation: Client will have a decrease in or will be free of ventricular arrhythmias.

Drug: lidocaine (Xylocaine HCL IV, Lido Pen Auto injector)

LIDDY LIDOCAINE

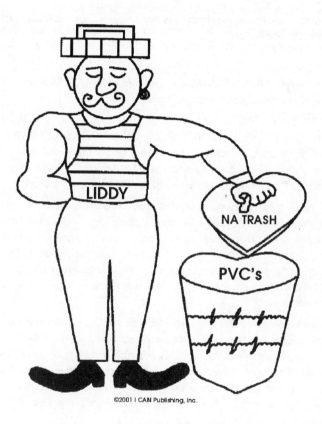

©2001 I CAN Publishing, Inc.

Liddy Lidocaine is the strongman that puts the lid on the sodium trash can of PVCs. This drug reduces sodium permeability, resulting in a decrease in ventricular arrhythmias and cardiac irritability.

Observe for undesirable effects, such as dizziness, drowsiness, and confusion.

AMIODARONE (CORDARONE)

Action: Antiarrhythmic (class III). Prolongs duration of action potential and effective refractory period, noncompetitive alpha and beta adrenergic inhibition; increases PR and QT intervals, decreases sinus rate, decreases peripheral vascular resistance.

Indication: Severe ventricular tachycardia, supraventricular tachycardia, (unlabeled use atrial fibrillation), ventricular fibrillation not controlled by first-line agents, cardiac arrest.

Warning: **HIGH ALERT DRUG** 2nd-, 3rd-degree AV block, bradycardia, severe sinus node dysfunction, neonates, infants.

Undesirable Effects: Headache, dizziness, fatigue, malaise, corneal microdeposits, Adult Respiratory Distress Syndrome (ARDS), Pulmonary Fibrosis, CHF, worsening of arrhythmias, bradycardia, hypotension. Liver function abnormalities: anorexia, constipation, nausea and vomiting. Toxic epidermal necrolysis: photosensitivity, hypothyroidism, ataxia, involuntary movements, peripheral neuropathy, poor coordination.

Other Specific Information: If taken with beta blockers or calcium channel blockers bradycardia may occur. Increased levels of digoxin (digoxin should be decreased by 50%), quinidine, procainamide, flecainide, disopyramide, phenytoin, theophylline, cyclosporine, dextromethorphan, methotrexate. Increased anticoagulant effects with warfarin (warfarin should be decreased by 33%–50%). Amiodarone effects may be increased if client is taking aloe, buckthorn bark/berry, cascara sagrada bark, rhubarb root, senna leaf/fruits.

Interventions: Assess I & O ratio: electrolytes (K, Na, Cl); liver function studies: AST, ALT, bilirubin, alk phosphatase. ECG continuously to determine drug effectiveness, measure PR, QRS, QT intervals, check for PVCs, other dysrhythmias, B/P continuously for hypotension, hypertension. Assess for rebound hypertension after 1–2 hr. Assess for ARDS, pulmonary fibrosis. Monitor pulse, respiratory rate, chest pain. Administer with meals if GI symptoms occur. If IV, administer via volumetric pump. Use an in line filter.

Education: Instruct to take drug as directed; avoid missed doses. Use sunscreens or stay out of sun to prevent burns. Report side effects. Advise that skin discoloration usually is reversible. If photophobia occurs, advise to wear sunglasses. Report unusual bleeding or bruising.

Staff Education: Do not confuse amiodarone (cordarone) with amrinone which is now called inamrinone (Inocor).

Evalutation: Client will have a decrease in ventricular tachycardia, supraventricular tachycardia or fibrillation.

Drugs: amiodarone (Cordarone, Pacerone)

CORDARONE

C oumadin must be decreased

O rdered for ventricular arrhythmias

R espiratoy Distress Syndrome (ARDS)—undesirable effect

D igoxin must be decreased

A taxia and dizziness—undesirable effects

R isk of bradycardia with beta
blockers and calcium channel blockers

O ral—administer with meals if GI distress
occurs

N ot confuse with amrinone

E valuate ECG for drug effectiveness

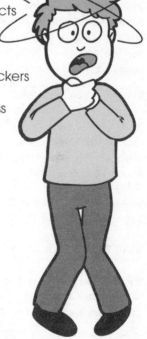

©2005 I CAN Publishing, Inc.

ADENOSINE

Action: Slows conduction through AV node, can interrupt reentry pathways through AV node, and can restore normal sinus rhythm in clients with supraventricular tachycardia (SVT).

Indications: SVT, as a diagnostic aid to assess myocardial perfusion defects in CAD.

Warnings: **HIGH ALERT DRUG**   Hypersensitivity, 2nd - or 3rd-degree heart block, AV block, sick sinus syndrome, atrial flutter, atrial fibrillation.

Undesirable Effects: Nausea, metallic taste, throat tightness, groin pressure; dyspnea, chest pressure, hyperventilation; lightheadedness, dizziness, arm tingling, numbness, apprehension, blurred vision, headache; chest pain, atrial tachydysrhythmias, sweating, palpitations, hypotension, facial flushing.

Other Specific Information: Increased effects of adenosine with dipyridamole. Decreased activity of adenosine when taken with theophylline or other methylxanthines (caffeine). An increased degree of heart block may occur when taken with carbamazepine. Possible ventricular fibrillation with digoxin. Smoking may increase tachycardia. May increase adenosine effect if taken with aloe, buckthorn bark/berry, cascara sagrada bark, rhubarb root, senna leaf/fruits. Decreased adenosine effect when taken with guarana.

Interventions: Assess I & O ratio, electrolytes (K, Na, Cl). Assess B/P, pulse, respiration, ECG intervals (PR, QRS, QT); check for transient dysrhythmias (PVCs, PACs, sinus tachycardia, AV block). Assess respiratory status: rhythm, rate, breath sounds. Assess for dizziness, confusion, psychosis, paresthesias, seizures. Treat overdose with defibrillation and vasopressor for hypotension.

Education: Advise to report facial flushing, dizziness, sweating, chest pain, or palpitations. Advise to rise slowly for a sitting or standing position to prevent orthostatic hypotension.

Staff Education: Do not confuse Adenocard with adenosine phosphate.

Evaluation: Client will have a normal sinus rhythm.

Drug: adenosine (Adenocard, Adenoscan)

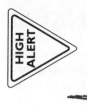

ADENOSINE

Don't administer

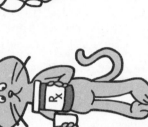

Caffine   Aloe   Theophylline   Smoking

©2005 I CAN Publishing, Inc.

These **CATS** will help you remember which agents to stay away from when taking these drugs. The first letter of each of these agents spells **CATS!**

CONCEPT: ANTIHYPERTENSIVE MEDICATIONS

Pressure (blood) monitor: Monitor blood pressure and pulse closely. A decrease in the blood pressure is an expected outcome, but it can also drop too much which can be unsafe.

Rise slowly to reduce orthostatic hypotension: Since orthostatic hypotension may occur, recommend the client to change positions slowly from recumbent to upright and dangle the feet from the edge of the bed to prevent dizziness. Recommend that the client not stand for long periods of time, not take hot showers, baths, or do strenuous exercise. Operating hazardous machinery or driving is not recommended until the response of the drugs has been determined since dizziness may occur. A Medic Alert bracelet or identification card should be carried in case of an emergency.

Eating must be considered (diet): The nonpharmacologic measure of sodium and fat reduction in the diet are strongly recommended.

Stay on medications: Clients have a tendency to stop a medication when they are feeling better. Instruct client regarding the importance of taking the medicine at the same time every day and taking it as prescribed. Recommend client stay away from over-the-counter cold, cough, or allergy medicines without first discussing with provider. Many are contraindicated with hypertension.

Skipping or stopping is a no-no: Review the importance of continuing drug even if undesirable effects occur; notify provider if effects occur. Abrupt discontinuation of these drugs may result in rebound hypertension.

Undesirable responses: Discuss with client that dizziness, drowsiness, and light-headedness may occur initially; inform provider of these symptoms. Each antihypertensive drug also has specific undesirable effects and should be reviewed with client. Instruct client to report these effects to provider and not to abruptly stop the drug.

Remind to exercise, no alcohol: Nonpharmacologic management of hypertension is important to emphasize. Regular exercise, weight reduction, behavior modification to promote relaxation, and moderate consumption of alcohol may assist in controlling hypertension.

Eliminate smoking; educate: The importance for smoking cessation should be emphasized to client. Instruct client and family members how to take a blood pressure reading and pulse. A record for the daily pressures should be recorded in a diary. Discuss the implications of hypertension and the long-term effects. Review the importance of periodic follow-up visits, so the blood pressure can be evaluated.

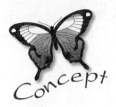
Concept

PRESSURE

P ressure (blood) monitor

R ise slowly to reduce orthostatic hypotension

E ating must be considered (diet)

S tay on medications

S kipping or stopping is a no-no

U ndesirable responses

R emind to exercise, ↓ alcohol

E liminate smoking; educate

©2001 I CAN Publishing, Inc.

ACE INHIBITORS

Action: Suppresses renin-angiotensin-aldosterone system; blocks conversion of angiotensin I to angiotensin II (a potent vasoconstrictor).

Indications: Hypertension, adjunctive therapy for CHF; reduces development of severe heart failure following MI in clients with impaired left ventricular function; protects against kidney failure in Type II diabetes.

Warnings: Renal or thyroid disease; severe salt/volume depletion; coronary insufficiency; leukemia.

Undesirable Effects: Gastric irritation, headache, dizziness, tachycardia, angioedema, cough, maculopapular rash, pruritus, infection, hyperkalemia.

Other Specific Information: Probenecid ↓elimination of ace inhibitors. NSAIDs may ↓hypotensive effects. ↑hypotensive effects with other antihypertensives. ↑K+ may occur with potassium-sparing diuretics, potassium supplements, or potassium containing salt substitutes.

Interventions: Obtain baseline and monitor serum/urine protein, BUN, creatinine, glucose, CBC with differential, potassium and sodium levels. First dose syncope may occur in those with CHF. Provide mouth care; alteration in taste may occur. (Refer to "**PRESSURE**".)

Education: Report any signs of infection, bruising, or bleeding. Captopril, moexipril, quinapril, and ramipril will have reduced absorption if given with food. 'Other ace inhibitors are not affected by food. Instruct not to use potassium supplements or any food or substance containing a large amount of potassium. (i.e., low-sodium milk, salt substitutes, etc.) (Refer to "**PRESSURE**".)

Evaluation: The blood pressure will return to normal limits without undesirable effects of these drugs.

Drugs: (*These drugs end in "pril".*) benaze**pril** (Lotension); capto**pril** (Capoten); enala**pril** (Vasotec); fosino**pril** (Monopril); lisino**pril** (Prinivil, Zestril); moexi**pril** (Univasc); perindo**pril** (Aceon); quina**pril** (Accupril); rami**pril** (Altace); trandola**pril** (Mavik)

PRIL SISTERS

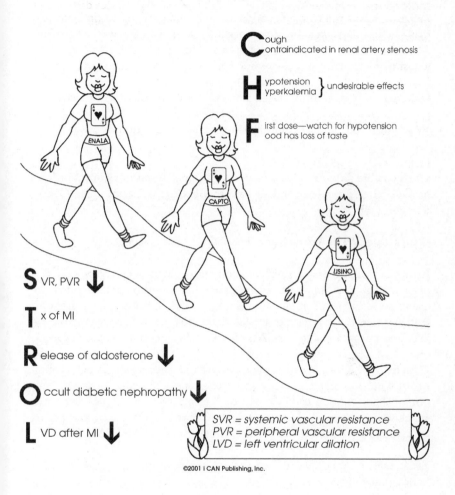

C ough
  ontraindicated in renal artery stenosis

H ypotension
  yperkalemia } undesirable effects

F irst dose—watch for hypotension
  ood has loss of taste

S VR, PVR ↓

T x of MI

R elease of aldosterone ↓

O ccult diabetic nephropathy ↓

L VD after MI ↓

SVR = systemic vascular resistance
PVR = peripheral vascular resistance
LVD = left ventricular dilation

©2001 i CAN Publishing, Inc.

The "Pril" sisters are taking a "strol" through the park to prevent cardiac problems. "STROL" will assist you in remebering the actions of ace inhibitors. "CHF" will help you in remembering some undesirable effects from these drugs.

ANGIOTENSIN II RECEPTOR BLOCKERS (ARBS)

Action: Blocks the binding of angiotensin II to the AT$_1$ receptor found in many tissues (*i.e., adrenal, vascular smooth muscle*). This blocks the vasoconstriction effect of the renin-angiotensin system as well as the release of aldosterone resulting in a decreased BP.

Indication: Hypertension. Used alone or with other antihypertensives.

Warnings: Renal/hepatic impairment; pregnancy/lactation; potassium supplements.

Undesirable Effects: Occasional—cough, upper respiratory infection, dizziness, diarrhea. Rare—back and leg pain, sinusitis, dyspepsia, insomnia. Overdosage— ↓ BP.

Other Specific Information: Phenobarbital may ↓ effects.

Interventions: Monitor renal function tests. Monitor BP and apical HR prior to each dose and on a regular basis. If hypotension occurs, place client in the supine position with feet slightly elevated. Maintain hydration. Administer without regard to meals. Assess for signs of upper respiratory infection, cough, and diarrhea. Assist with ambulation if dizziness occurs.

Education: Report any signs of an infection. Do not take cold preparations or nasal decongestants. Caution about exercising during hot weather due to potential dehydration and hypotension. Use a barrier method of birth control. Instruct not to use potassium supplements or any food containing large amounts of potassium (i.e., salt substitutes). (Refer to "**PRESSURE**".)

Evaluation: Client's blood pressure will return to normal range with no undesirable effects.

Drugs: (*These drugs end in "sartan".*) cande**sartan** (Atacand); epro**sartan** (Teveten); irbe**sartan** (Avapro); lo**sartan** (Cozaar); telmi**sartan** (Micardis); val**sartan** (Diovan)

SARTAN SISTERS

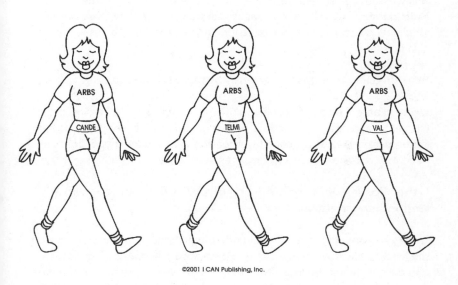

©2001 I CAN Publishing, Inc.

A dminister without regard to meals

R enal function tests—review

B locks vasoconstriction effect of renin—angiotensin system

S alt substitution or potassium supplements—do not use

Cande, Telmi, and Val SARTAN are working to reduce hypertension.

ALPHA ADRENERGIC BLOCKERS

Action: Blocks alpha$_1$ adrenergic receptors resulting in vasodilation of arteries and veins. ↓ peripheral vascular resistance; relaxes smooth muscle of bladder/prostate.

Indications: Hypertension (terazosin, doxazosin). Prazosin has been used as adjunct therapy for CHF. Doxazosin and terazosin may be used for benign prostatic hyperplasia.

Warnings: Renal disease. Elderly may be more sensitive to drug.

Undesirable Effects: Dizziness, drowsiness, weakness, depression; palpitations, tachycardia, orthostatic hypotension; urinary frequency, dry mouth; impotence. First-dose syncope (hypotension with sudden loss of consciousness) may occur between 2–6 hrs. after initial dose.

Other Specific Information: ↑ hypotensive effect with other antihypertensives, nitrates, alcohol.

Interventions: Monitor BP frequently and protect from falling/injury after the first dose and with each ↑ due to first-dose syncope. If initial dose or ↑ in dose is during the day, client must remain recumbent for 3–4 hours. Assess BP and HR immediately before each dose. Assist with ambulating if client is dizzy. (Refer to "**PRESSURE**".)

Education: Caution that the first-dose syncope may occur, and implement safety precautions. Report if edema is present in the AM. Sugarless gum, sips of tepid water, etc. may relieve dry mouth. (Refer to "**PRESSURE**".)

Evaluation: Client's blood pressure will remain in normal limits with no undesirable effects from the medications.

Drugs: doxazo**sin** (Cardura); prazo**sin** (Minipress); terazo**sin** (Hytrin)

MINI'S SINS

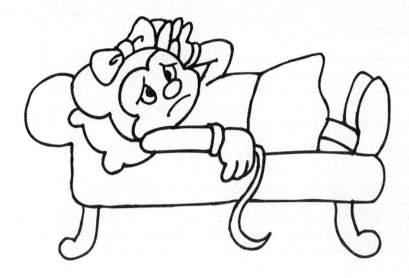

©2001 I CAN Publishing, Inc.

S yncope
  exual dysfunction

I ncreased drowsiness, orthostatic hypotension, HR

N eed to be recumbent for 3–4 hours after initial dose

Mini's "SINS" (minipress) are undesireable effects of Alpha Adrenergic Blockers. These medications end in **SIN**.

BETA-ADRENERGIC BLOCKERS

Action: Binds to beta 1–(cardiac) and/or beta 2–(lungs) adrenergic receptor sites that prevents the release of catecholamine. Refer to page 58 to assist with this information. The "**LOL**" Team will also assist you in recalling the actions of this category. They include a ↓ in contractility, ↓ renin release, and ↓ in the sympathetic output .

Indications: Hypertension, angina, MI; migraine headaches, situational anxiety; thyrotoxic storm/crisis; upper GI bleed; familial (essential) tremors; and assists in treatment of dysrrhythmias.

Warnings: COPD, asthma, CHF, sinus bradycardia, heart block > first degree; diabetes mellitus.

Undesirable Effects: Refer to " **BLOCKER**" to assist in recalling these effects (page 59).

Other Specific Information: Anticholinergics ↑absorption. Antacids ↓ absorption. ↑risk for bradycardia when used concurrently with cardiac glycosides and calcium channel blockers. ↑hypotensive effects when given with diuretics. Sudden discontinuing may cause refractory hypertension. *(Refer to a Drug Handbook for reviewing the numerous drug-drug interactions which may occur.)*

Interventions: Monitor blood sugar closely in clients with diabetes. Monitor triglyceride and cholesterol level (LDL). Monitor BP and pulse prior to administering. If pulse is < 60 or SBP < 90, withhold and notify provider of health care. Monitor any change in the cardiac rhythm or any signs of CHF. (Refer to "**PRESSURE**".)

Education: Instruct client regarding self assessment of pulse, character, and rhythm; signs and symptoms of CHF. Avoid heat, excessive exercise, hot showers, baths and hot tubs. (Refer to "**PRESSURE**".)

Evaluation: The blood pressure will return to normal limits. If given for arrhythmias, the ECG will record a normal sinus rhythm.

Drugs: *(These drugs end in "lol".)* ***Cardioselective (Beta 1 receptors):*** acebuto**lol** (Sectral), ateno**lol** (Tenormin), betaxo**lol** (Kerlone), bisopro**lol** (Zebeta), esmo**lol** (Brevibloc), metopro**lol** (Lopressor, Toprol XL); ***Nonselective (Beta 1 and Beta 2 receptors):*** carteo**lol** (Cartrol); carvedi**lol** (Coreg); labeta**lol** (Normodyne); nado**lol** (Corgard); penbuto**lol** (Levotol); pindo**lol** (Visken); proprano**lol** (Inderal); sota**lol** (Betapace); timo**lol** (Blocadren)

For Beta 2 Selective Drugs see MAX AIR

THE "LOL" TEAM

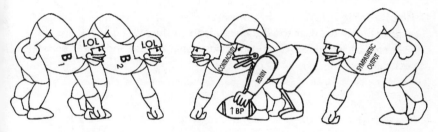

©2001 I CAN Publishing, Inc.

The **"LOL"** team blocks hypertension by "blocking" (decreasing) the contractility in the heart, the renin release from the kidneys, and the sympathetic output from the vasomotor center of the brain.

BETA BLOCKER ACTIONS

B_1 **BLOCKERS AFFECT** [heart icon with 1]

Beta$_1$ Blockers affect the Beta$_1$ receptors in the heart. They ↓ the excitability, cardiac workload, O_2 consumption, renin release and lower blood pressure

B_2 **BLOCKERS AFFECT** [lung icon with 2]

©2001 I CAN PUBLISHING, INC.

Beta$_2$ Blockers stimulate the beta receptors in the lung, relax bronchial smooth muscle, ↑ vital capacity, and ↓ airway resistance. Higher doses may cause undesirable cardiac effects.

BLOCKER

BRADYCARDIA
BLOOD PRESSURE—TOO LOW
BRONCHIAL CONSTRICTION
BLOOD SUGAR—MASKS LOW

©2005 I CAN Publishing, Inc.

"BLOCKER" outlines undesirable effects of Beta Blockers.

CALCIUM CHANNEL BLOCKERS

Action: Blocks calcium access to the cells causing a ↓ in contractility, ↓ arteriolar constriction, ↓ PVR, and ↓ BP.

Indications: Hypertension; vasospastic angina; classic chronic stable angina; atrial fibrillation or flutter; migraine headaches. **Nimodipine** is selective for cerebral arteries. **Bepridil** prevents coronary artery spasm making it an agent for chronic stable angina. **These 2 medications are not indicated for hypertension.**

Warnings: Severe CHF; 2nd or 3rd degree AV block; sick sinus syndrome; SBP < 90 mm Hg; bradycardia; aortic stenosis; caution in the elderly client due to long half-life.

Undesirable Effects: Hypotension, headache, dizziness; atrioventricular block; worsens CHF; peripheral edema; constipation. (*Refer to image on next page!*)

Other Specific Information: Beta-adrenergic blockers may ↑ cardiac depression when given with calcium channel blockers. ↑ serum levels of digoxin, carbamazepine, and quinidine result when given with calcium channel blockers. ↑ serum levels when administered with cimetidine or ranitidine.

Interventions: Monitor hepatic and renal function studies. Monitor ECG and avoid giving when heart blocks are present. During bepridil therapy, periodic K+ levels may be required. Have emergency equipment available with IV administration. Protect drug from light and moisture. Position client to decrease peripheral edema. (Refer to "**PRESSURE**".)

Education: Instruct to ↑ dietary fiber, fluid intake, and exercise. Avoid overexertion when anginal pain is relieved. Encourage to take with meals or milk. Recommend client not to chew or crush sustained-release. (Refer to "**PRESSURE**".)

Evaluation: The blood pressure will be within normal limits. There will be a normal sinus rhythm on the ECG. If administered for angina or headaches, there will be a decrease in the symptoms.

Drugs: amlodipine (Norvasc); bepridil (Vascor); diltiazem (Cardizem); felodipine (Plendil) SR; isradipine (DynaCirc) SR; nicardipine (Cardene) SR; nifedipine (Procardia) SR; nimodipine (Nimotop); nisoldipine (Sular); verapamil (Isoptin, Calan)

SR = Sustained release

CALCIUM CHANNEL BLOCKERS

"DON'T GIVE A FLIP PILLS"

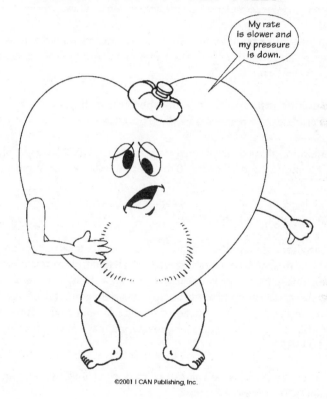

©2001 I CAN Publishing, Inc.

Major undesirable effects of calcium channel blockers include: headache (most common), hypotension, syncope, peripheral edema, bradycardia and constipation. These clients "don't give a flip" at times (syncope) or from just feeling "blah" from the other undesirable effects.

CENTRAL ALPHA₂ AGONISTS

Action: Decreases the release of adrenergic hormones from the brain, resulting in a ↓ in the peripheral vascular resistance and blood pressure.

Indications: Hypertension (stepped-care approach, step 2 drug).

Warnings: Acute hepatitis; active cirrhosis. Recent MI; severe coronary artery insufficiency; cerebrovascular disease; chronic renal failure.

Undesirable Effects: Transient drowsiness, headache, weakness during initial therapy. Dry mouth, constipation, hypotension, bradycardia, occasional edema, or weight gain.

Other Specific Information: ↓ antihypertensive effects with TCAs (imipramine). Paradoxical hypertension with propranolol.

Interventions: Monitor liver/renal function tests, CBC, baseline BP, P, and weights. Monitor BP and VS every 30 minutes until stable during initial therapy. Rapid ↑ in BP and symptoms of sympathetic over activity (i.e., ↑ pulse, tremor agitation, and anxiety) may occur. Catapres may be given to rapidly ↓ BP in some hypertensive emergencies.

Education: Recommend the last dose of the day be taken at bedtime. Give medication with snack. Thorough effect of oral administration may take 2–3 days. Weigh daily. Notify provider if weight gain > 4 lbs. in 1 week. Drowsiness disappears during continued therapy. Sugarless gum, sips of tepid water may relieve dry mouth. Give diuretic if needed. If need to discontinue, taper dose gradually over more than one week. Urine may darken in color. (Refer to "**PRESSURE**".)

Evaluation: Blood pressure will return to normal limits with no undesirable effects from the medications.

Drugs: clonidine (Catapres); guanabenz (Wytensin); guanfacine (Tenex); methyldopa (Aldomet)

CATAPRES

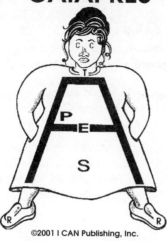

©2001 I CAN Publishing, Inc.

C is at her eyes because the adrenergic hormone is released from the brain.

A is at her nose because the risk factors of hypotension, hepatotoxicity and hemolytic anemia are as clear as the nose on her face.

T is at her chin as it drops with transient drowsiness.

A is "body-wide" because arterial pressure all over the body is lowered.

P indicates paradoxical hypertension with propranolol.

R is at her baseline feet to remind you to record baseline vital signs.

E on her belt may expand because she may have a weight gain; evaluate her liver.

S is tapered down her dress because the drugs should be slowly tapered down and not stopped suddenly.

Catapres, a commonly used antihypertensive drug is the name of our image to review the actions of central alpha$_2$ agonists. Studies show that women of color have increased risk of hypertension. See that the letters in Catapres are placed on her image.

VASODILATORS

Action: Direct relaxation of vascular smooth muscle, producing vasodilation of arterioles which decreases afterload.

Indications: Hypertension.

Warnings: Coronary artery disease, rheumatic heart disease, hydralazine-lupus, pregnancy, impaired renal function, CVA.

Undesirable Effects: Headache, dizziness; anorexia, nausea, vomiting, diarrhea; palpitations, tachycardia, hypotension, occasional postural hypotension; edema and/or weight gain (drugs can cause sodium and water retention); flushing; nasal congestion. Lupus-like reaction (fever, facial rash, muscle and joint ache, splenomegaly).

Other Specific Information: ↑ hypotensive effects with antihypertensives, beta blockers, and diuretics.

Interventions: Monitor BP, heart rate, daily weight, CBC, ANA titers, renal function tests, urinalysis. (Refer to "**PRESSURE**".)

Education: Instruct how to take heart rate. If rate is > 20 beats per minute over normal, notify provider. Report a 5 lb. weight gain. Monitor and report muscle and joint aches, fever (lupus-like reaction). Monitor bowel activity. Take with meals; for nausea eat unsalted crackers or dry toast. Report peripheral edema of hands and feet. Lie down if dizzy. (Refer to "**PRESSURE**".)

Evaluation: Client's BP will return to normal range with no undesirable effects.

Drugs: hydralazine (Apresoline); minoxidil (Loniten)

DILLY DILATOR

D irectly acts on vascular smooth muscle, causing vasodilation

I ncreases renal and cerebral blood flow

L upus-like reaction (fever, facial rash, muscle and joint ache, splenomegaly—U E)

A ssess for peripheral edema of hands and feet

T ake with food

O ther U E—headache, dizziness, anorexia, tachycardia, hypotension

R eview BP

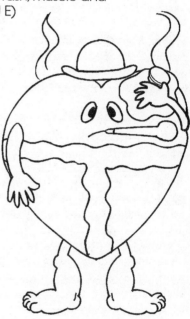

©2001 I CAN Publishing, Inc.

Dilly Dilator's heart vessels are enlarged to allow more O_2 to the heart muscle. If they become too dilated he will have hypotension on rising, headache, and diarrhea. His temperature may rise due to a "lupus-like" reaction.

CONCEPT: DIURETICS

Diet: Instruct client to eat a low sodium diet and a diet rich in potassium. Clients taking potassium-sparing diuretics should not eat a diet rich in potassium!

Intake and Output, daily weight: These are outcomes that can assist in evaluating the effects of the drugs. There should be an increase in the urine output. Hard candy, sips of water, sugarless gum, etc. may be effective if client has a dry mouth.

Undesirable effects: fluid and electrolyte imbalance: Monitor the fluid and electrolytes while a client is taking diuretics and report changes to provider. *Hypovolemia:* ↑ HR with weak pulse, ↑ respirations, ↓ B/P, and ↓ output. *Hypokalemia:* abnormal ECG, orthostatic hypotension, flaccid paralysis, and weakness. *Hyperkalemia:* nausea, diarrhea, abnormal ECG, confusion, muscle weakness, tingling in the extremities, paresthesia, dyspnea, and fatigue. (concern with potassium-sparing diuretic) (Therapeutic: 3.5–5.0 mEq/L). *Hyponatremia:* lethargy, disorientation, muscle tenseness, seizures, coma (Therapeutic: 135–145mEq/L)

Review HR and BP: Due to potential hypovolemia, monitor the HR and BP. If client is taking digoxin, evaluate for signs of hypokalemia due to risk of digoxin toxicity.

Elderly–CAREFUL: Due to physiological changes in this population, an accurate assessment of fluid, electrolytes, and BP is important. Evaluate adequate renal function by checking the creatinine clearance in the elderly.

Take with or after meals and in AM: Instruct client to take with or after meals if GI distress occurs. Nausea and vomiting may be a result of electrolyte disturbance. Administering the diuretics early in the day will help avoid nocturia.

Increase risk of orthostatic hypotension: Due to this risk, instruct client to change positions slowly especially when rising.

Cancel alcohol: Alcohol products need to be canceled due to the diuresing effect and the risk of decreasing the blood pressure too much.

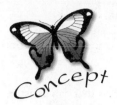
Concept

DIURETIC

D iet— ↑ K+ for all except aldactone

I ntake & output, daily weight

U ndesirable effects: fluid & electrolyte imbalance

R eview HR, BP, and electrolytes

E LDERLY—careful
evening dose not recommended

T ake with or after meals and in AM

I ncrease risk of orthostatic hypotension; move slowly

C ancel alcohol, cigarettes

©2001 I CAN Publishing, Inc.

LOOP DIURETICS

Action: Inhibits sodium, chloride, and water reabsorption in the proximal portion of the ascending loop of Henle.

Indications: Edema associated with congestive heart failure, cirrhosis with ascites, or renal dysfunction. Furosemide for hypertension or in combination with other antihypertensive medications.

Warnings: Hypokalemia, hypersensitivity to sulfonamides or loop diuretics; renal/hepatic dysfunction; gout; diabetes.

Undesirable Effects: Hyponatremia, hypokalemia, hypocalcemia, hypomag-nesemia, hypochloremic alkalosis, hyperglycemia, and hyperuricemia. (*Remember everything is decreased except the glucose and uric acid!*) Hypotension; blurred vision, headaches, dizziness, lightheadedness; anorexia, nausea, diarrhea; dehydration, muscle cramp, ototoxicity. Furosemide and ethacrynic acid may cause leukopenia and photosensitivity.

Other Specific Information: ↑ in digitalis and lithium toxicity. ↓ K+ with corticosteroids, and some penicillins. ↓ effects of antiocoagulants. Avoid amphotericin B, nephrotoxic, or other ototoxic medications.

Interventions: Monitor serum glucose, and electrolytes. (Refer to "**DIURETIC**".)

Education: Report changes in hearing, irritability, vomiting, anorexia, nausea, diarrhea, twitching, or tetany. (Refer to "**DIURETIC**".)

Evaluation: Client's blood pressure and edema will decrease and remain within normal range.

Drugs: bumetanide (Bumex); ethacrynic acid (Edecrin); furosemide (Lasix); torsemide (Demadex)

LOU LA BELL

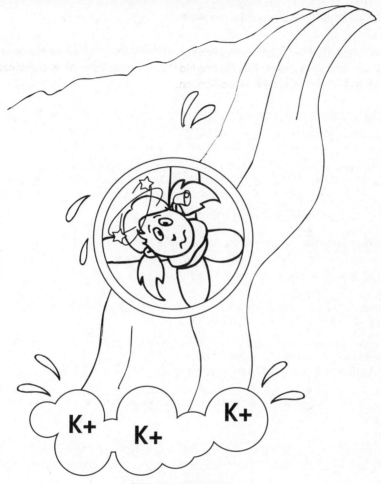

©2001 I CAN Publishing, Inc.

Lou La Bell goes spinning over the falls because she has lost so much fluid from diuresing. Her ears are ringing and she is dizzy from a decrease in her blood pressure. She has lost potassium in the falls. Loop diuretics act in the ascending loop of Henle and one common drug is Lasix.

Remember, Thiazides at the distal tubule (major differences between undesirable effects between Thiazides and Loops is that Loops may cause ototoxicity and hypocalcemia).

THIAZIDES

Action: Increases urine output by inhibiting reabsorption of sodium, chloride, and water in the distal portion of the ascending Loop of Henle.

Indications: Edema associated with congestive heart failure, cirrhosis with ascites, and some types of renal impairment (*i.e., acute glomerulonephritis, and nephrotic syndrome*). Hypertension.

Warnings: Hypokalemia; hypersensitivity to sulfonamides or thiazide diuretics; renal/hepatic dysfunction. Caution with the elderly, clients with diabetes mellitus, gout, or history of lupus erythematosus.

Undesirable effects: Hypokalemia; hyponatremia; hyperuricemia; hypercalcemia; hyperglycemia. Orthostatic hypotension, syncope; anorexia, nausea, or vomiting; dehydration; photosensitivity.

Other Specific Information: ↑ risk of digitalis (if hypokalemia present) and lithium toxicity. ↑ loss of potassium when taking corticosteroids and some penicillins. ↓ effects of antidiabetic agents.

Interventions: Check for allergies to sulfonamides. Monitor serum glucose, and K+ levels. (Refer to "**DIURETIC**".)

Education: Instruct to discontinue thiazides prior to parathyroid function tests due to the altered calcium levels. (Refer to "**DIURETIC**".)

Evaluation: Client's blood pressure and edema will be ↓ and remain within normal range.

Drugs: chlorothiazide (Diuril); chlorthalidone (Hygroton); hydrochlorothiazide (Esidrix, HCTZ, HydroDiuril); indapamide (Lozol); metolazone (Zaroxolyn)

THIAZIDE DIURETICS
"LOU LA BELL"

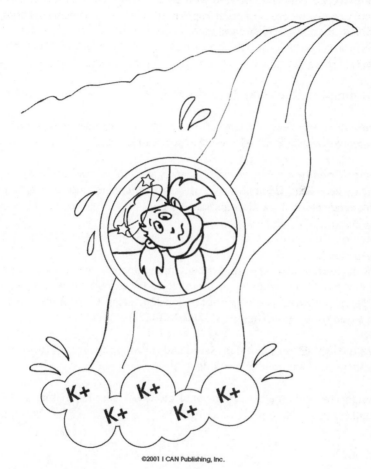

K+ K+ K+ K+ K+

©2001 I CAN Publishing, Inc.

Lou La Bell is experiencing syncope, dehydration (from all the diuresing "waterfall"), electrolyte imbalance (hypokalemia) and orthostatic hypotension from the thiazide diuretics.

Thiazides act in the distal tubule. Major differences from the loop diuretics are calcium may be high (rhymes with thigh[azide]) and the client experiences no ototoxicity with thiazide diuretics.

POTASSIUM SPARING DIURETICS

Action: Promotes excretion of sodium and water, but retains potassium in the distal renal tubule.

Indications: Used with loop or thiazide diuretics in treating CHF and hypertension. Diuretic induced hypokalemia. Steroid-induced edema. Hyperaldosteronism.

Warnings: Impaired renal functions; PIH; hyperkalemia; diabetes mellitus.

Undesirable Effects: Nausea, diarrhea, dizziness, headache, dry mouth, rash, photosensitivity. ↑ K+ levels result in peaked T waves on ECG.

Other Specific Information: ↑ digitalis and lithium toxicity. ↑ K+ levels when taken with ACE inhibitors, potassium containing medications, or potassium supplements. ↓ anticoagulant effects.

Interventions: Monitor K+ and digitalis levels. (Refer to "**DIURETIC**".)

Education: Inform client that maximum hypotensive effect may not be seen for 2 weeks. Counsel client to avoid citrus juices, colas, milk low in sodium, some salt substitutes, or other potassium supplements. Monitor for ↑ K+ during blood transfusion. (Refer to "**DIURETIC**".)

Evaluation: Client's blood pressure and serum potassium will remain within normal limits; edema will decrease.

Drugs: amiloride (Midamor); spironolactone (Aldactone); triamterene (Dyrenium)

ALAN ALDACTONE

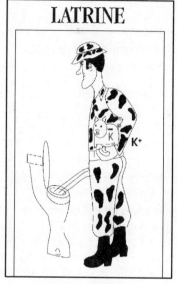

LATRINE

©2001 I CAN Publishing, Inc.

L ow Na^+

E levated T waves from ↑K^+

A granulocytosis with triamterene

K $^+$ level must be monitored

Alan Aldactone is at the latrine taking a leak and getting rid of the extra volume that's increasing his blood pressure. Alan is holding his piggy bank with K^+ on it, as aldactone helps in saving potassium.

OSMOTIC DIURETICS

Action: Increases osmotic pressure of glomerular filtrate, thus preventing reabsorption of water. Increases excretion of sodium and chloride.

Indications: Oliguria, edema, increased intracranial pressure; increased intracocular pressure; treat certain drug toxicities.

Warnings: Heart failure, renal failure, hypertension, pulmonary edema due to transient increase in blood pressure; intracranial hemorrhage; severe dehydration. Serum osmolality > 310–320 mOsm/kg is contraindicated.

Undesirable Effects: Dry mouth, thirst, nausea, vomiting, blurred vision, headache, dizziness. Cellular dehydration; fluid and electrolyte imbalance; pulmonary edema.

Other Specific Information: May ↑ Digitalis toxicity.

Interventions: Monitor renal function tests, serum and urine K+ and Na+ levels, CVP, and vital signs. Watch for rapid ↑ in BP and symptoms of sympathetic overactivity (i.e., ↑ heart rate, tremor, and agitation). Solutions given IV only via an in line filter. IV solution may crystallize; re-dissolve before infusing by warming bottle. Never give solutions with undissolved crystals. (Refer to "**DIURETIC**".)

Education: Advise client that glycerin and isosorbide are for the reduction of intraocular pressure and should be monitored by the provider of care frequently. (Refer to "**DIURETIC**".)

Evaluation: Intracranial or intraocular pressure should be reduced. If given for renal failure, diuresing should occur with an improvement in the BUN and serum creatinie values.

Drugs: glycerin (Osmoglyn); isosorbide (Ismotic); mannitol (Osmitrol); urea (Ureaphil)

BUSTER BRAIN MAN

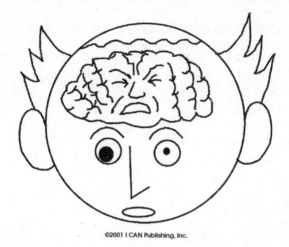

©2001 I CAN Publishing, Inc.

O liguira, edema, ↑ ICP—indications

S tops reabsorption of water

M annitol

O utput of urine, electrolytes—monitor

T issue dehydration—U E

I ncreased frequency/volume of urination

C irculatory overload—U E

Buster Brain Man is feeling the squeeze from too much fluid in the brain. He can't think, he can't blink, and he may sink without an osmotic diuretic. Mannitol will reduce this cerebral edema.

CONCEPT: ANTICOAGULANTS

This category is commonly referred to as anticoagulants or "blood thinners". While they do not actually **"thin"** the blood, they work on different factors in the blood to decrease its ability to clot. This decrease in clotting prevents harmful clots from forming in the vessels. They also can interfere or inhibit platelet aggregation which in turn prevents the clots from forming or attaching to the vessels. Despite the type of action they have, all blood viscosity reducing agents are considered **HIGH ALERT** medications and safeguards at practice sites should be adopted.

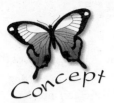

ANTICOAGULANTS

Concept

T hese belong to class of meds called anticoagulants

H ospitalization required for IV Heparin

I nform other physicians (dentists, surgeons, etc.) that client is taking these meds

N ote an increase in bruising or bleeding tendencies

B eware of mixing with herbal supplements

L ook for nose bleeds—this may be the first sign that dose is too high

O ral drugs require frequent blood test to monitor

O ften prescribed with heart valve replacements

D on't take in large amounts of vitamin K (fish liver, spinach, cabbage, etc.)

©2005 I CAN Publishing, Inc.

ANTICOAGULANT: WARFARIN

Action: Interferes with the hepatic synthesis of vitamin K-clotting factors (II, VII, IX, and X).

Indications: Prevents or slows extension of a blood clot.

Undesirable Effects: Anorexia, nausea, diarrhea; rash; bleeding, hematuria, thrombocytopenia, hemorrhage.

Warnings: Pregnancy; hemorrhagic tendencies such as hemophilia, thrombocytopenia purpura, leukemia; peptic ulcer; cerebral vascular accident (CVA); severe renal or hepatic disease.

Other Specific Information: Foods—↑ effectiveness (i.e. asparagus, cabbage, cauliflower, turnip greens, and other green leafy vegetables). Drugs—↑ effectiveness: **G**lucocorticosteroids, **A**lcohol, **S**alicylate (**GAS**). Drugs ↓ effectiveness: **R**ifampin, **O**ral contraceptives, **P**henytoin, **E**strogen (**ROPE**). ↑ risk of bleeding with chamomile, garlic, ginger, ginkgo, and ginseng therapy. There are numerous interactions. (*Refer to a Drug Handbook.*)

Interventions: "**CORA**" on the next page will help you remember 4 major interventions. Anticoagulant effects may be reversed by vitamin K injections. Check all drugs for potential drug-drug interactions.

Education: Evaluation of PT/INR will be required to regulate dosage; report any unusual bleeding. Review a diet low in vitamin K. Wear a medical identification card or jewelry (Medic Alert). Always advise other providers (i.e., dentists, surgeon, etc.) of medication; no strenuous activities (skydiving, long distance running, football); no OTC medication without provider approval.

Evaluation: PT will have a value of 1.5 to 2.5 times the control value in seconds; the INR will be 2–3. The client will have no signs or symptoms of bleeding.

Drug: warfarin (Coumadin)

CORA COUMADIN

HIGH
ALERT

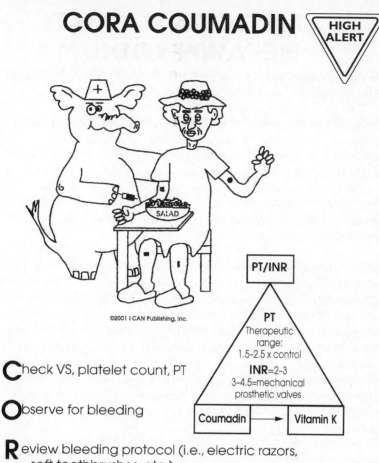

©2001 I CAN Publishing, Inc.

PT/INR

PT
Therapeutic
range:
1.5–2.5 x control

INR=2–3
3–4.5=mechanical
prosthetic valves

| Coumadin | → | Vitamin K |

Check VS, platelet count, PT

Observe for bleeding

Review bleeding protocol (i.e., electric razors,
soft toothbrushes, etc.)

Avoid ASA, may use acetaminophen

Cora Coumadin is having her blood drawn for coagulation levels. If her
PT is > 1.5–2.5 x the control, she may experience excessive bruising and
have bloody stools. Foods high in vitamin K (such as green leafy vegetables)
should be avoided since they will increase the risk of clotting.

ANTICOAGULANT: HEPARIN SODIUM

Action: Combines with antithrombin III to retard thrombin activity. Low-molecular-weight heparin blocks factor Xa, factor IIa.

Indications: Thrombosis. Reduces risk of myocardial infarction (MI), CVA, clots associated with atrial fibrillation; pulmonary embolism.

Warnings: Hypersensitivity to heparin; severe thrombocytopenia; uncontrolled bleeding; ulcers or any risk of hemorrhage; liver or renal disease.

Undesirable Effects: Hemorrhagic tendencies: hematuria, bleeding gums, frank hemorrhage.

Other Specific Information: ↑ effect with aspirin, alcohol, and antibiotics. ↓ effect with digoxin (Lanoxin), antihistamines, and nitroglycerin products. ↑ risk of bleeding with chamomile, garlic, ginger, ginkgo, and ginseng therapy.

Interventions: Monitor PTT (usually 1.5–2.5 times control values) and platelet count. Monitor for signs of unusual bleeding (petechiae, hematuria, GI bleeding, gum bleeding). Initiate bleeding protocol measures (use electric razors, hold pressure for 5 minutes with venipunctures, soft toothbrushes). Monitor IV site carefully. Heparin has short half life, therefore, with discontinuation, PTT will usually return to baseline within 1–2 hours. Have protamine sulfate available as an antidote.

Education: Explain bleeding protocol precautions; explain the need for several PTT evaluations; teach signs of unusual bleeding; avoid activities with risk of injury; caution with sharp utensils while cooking or eating. Avoid salicylates or any OTC medication without approval from provider. Wear identification that notes anticoagulant therapy. Inform provider of therapy prior to surgical procedure.

Evaluation: The client's PTT will show values 1.5–2.5 times the control value in seconds, and there will be no signs or symptoms of bleeding or thrombus formation.

Drugs: Heparin Sodium (Heparin); **Low-Molecular-Weight Heparins:** ardeparin (Normiflo); dalteparin (Fragmin); danaparoid (Orgaran); enoxaparin (Lovenox)

HARRY HEPARIN

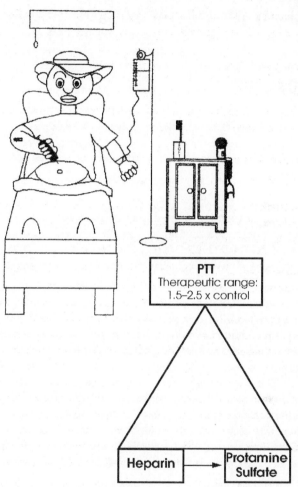

©2001 I CAN Publishing, Inc.

Harry Heparin is getting his anticoagulant IV or SubQ in the abdomen. His soft toothbrush will help keep gums from bleeding and his electric razor will keep him from bleeding when he shaves. Even the band-aid when pulled off his arm may cause a big bruise. If Harry's PTT is > 1.5–2.5 x control, he may bruise and bleed too freely.

ANTICOAGULANT: ENOXAPARIN
(Low molecular weight heparin)

Action: Anticoagulant, antithrombotic. Prevents conversion of fibrinogen to fibrin and prothrombin to thrombin by enhancing inhibitory effects of antithrombin III; produces higher ratio of anti-factor Xa to IIa

Indications: Prevention of deep-vein thrombosis, pulmonary emboli in hip and knee replacement

Warnings: **HIGH ALERT DRUG**   Hypersensitivity to drug, heparin, or pork; hemophilia, leukemia with bleeding, peptic ulcer disease, thrombocytopenic purpura, heparin - induced thrombocytopenia, clients with prosthetic heart valves.

Undesirable Effects: Fever, confusion, nausea, edema, hypochromic anemia, thrombo-cytopenia, bleeding, cardiac toxicity, ecchymosis.

Other Specific Information: Increased action of enoxaparin: anticoagulants, salicy-lates, NSAIDs, antiplatelets. Increased hypoprothrombinemia: plicamycin, valproic acid. **DO NOT MIX WITH OTHER DRUGS OR INFUSION FLUIDS.** Increased risk of bleeding when taken with bromelain, cinchona bark, garlic ginger, ginkgo, and ginseng.

Interventions: Assess blood studies (i.e., Hct, CBC, coagulation studies, platelets, occult blood in stools), anti-factor Xa; thrombocytopenia may occur. Assess for bleeding: gums, petechiae, ecchymosis, black tarry stools, hematuria; notify prescriber. Assess for neu-rologic symptoms in clients who have received spinal anesthesia. Administer only after screening for bleeding disorders. **SC only (do not aspirate or massage); do not give IM,** begin 2 hrs prior to surgery, do not aspirate, rotate sites, do not expel bubble from syringe prior to administration. Insert whole length of needle into skin fold held with thumb and forefinger. Administer only this drug when ordered; not interchangeable with heparin. Leave vascular access sheath in place for 6 hr after dose, then give next dose 6 hr after sheath removal. Avoid all IM injections that my cause bleeding. Treatment of overdose should be Protamine Sulfate; dose should equal dose of enoxaparin.

Education: Instruct client to use soft-bristle toothbrush to avoid bleeding gums, to use electric razor. Report any signs of bleeding: gums, under skin, urine, stools. Avoid over the counter drugs containing aspirin.

Staff Education: Do not confuse enoxaparin with enoxacin or Lovenox with Lotronex.

Evaluation: Client will not experience any deep vein thrombosis and will have a thera-peutic response.

Drugs: enoxaparin (Lovenox)

ENOXAPARIN "LOVENOX"

HIGH ALERT

L ow molecular weight

O rthopedic surgeries

D **V** T prophylaxis, immobility, stints, cardiac surgeries
—indicators

L **E** ave bubble in syringe

N ever by IM, only subcutaneous—give within 2 hours
of preop abdominal surgery and 12 hours of
knee surgery

N **O** rubbing after administered, no aspiration, no mixing with
other drugs

X out for pork allergies,
heparin allergies; PUD;
leukemia

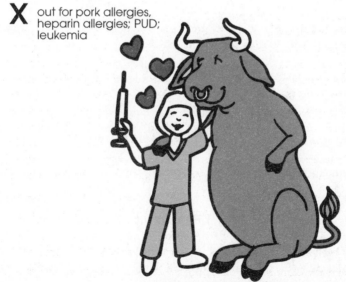

©2005 I CAN Publishing, Inc.

"Love an ox" by initiating bleeding protocols, having protamine sulfate on hand for antidote and monitoring coagulation studies.

ANTIPLATELET: ASPIRIN

Action: Platelet aggregation inhibitor; inhibits platelet synthesis of thromboxane A_2, a vasoconstrictor and inducer of platelet aggregation. This occurs at low doses and lasts for 8 days (life of the platelet).

Indications: TIAs; CVAs with a history of TIA due to fibrin platelet emboli. Reduces risk of death from MI in clients with a history of infarction or unstable angina. (Refer to **NSAIDs.**)

Warnings: Allergy to salicylates or NSAIDs. Bleeding disorders, renal or hepatic disorders, chickenpox, influenza (risk of Reye's in syndrome in children), pregnancy, lactation.

Undesirable Effects: GI discomfort, bleeding, dizziness, tinnitus. (Refer to **NSAIDs.**)

Other Specific Information: ↑risk of bleeding with anticoagulants, thrombolytics. ↑risk of GI ulceration with alcohol, NSAIDs, phenylbutazone, steroids.

Interventions: Monitor liver and renal function tests, CBC, clotting times, stool guaiac, blood drug levels, and vital signs.

Education: Instruct to take drug with food and a full glass of water. Do not crush and do not chew sustained-release preparations. Use only as recommended. Review undesirable effects and the importance of reporting them to the provider. Initiate safety precautions to keep out of children's reach since it can be very dangerous. (Refer to **NSAIDs.**)

Evaluation: Client will experience no thrombotic episodes, such as a stroke.

Drugs: aspirin (Bayer, Bufferin, Ecotrin); *Other antiplatelet drugs are listed below; however, there are numerous differences between each drug. (Refer to Drug Handbook.)* abciximab (ReoPro); cilostazol (Pletal); clopidogrel (Plavix); dipyridamole (Persantine); eptifibatide (Integrilin); sulfinpyrazone (Anturane); ticlopidine (Ticlid); tirofiban (Aggrastat)

ANNIE ASPIRIN

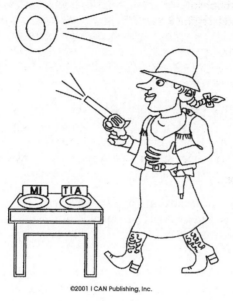

©2001 I CAN Publishing, Inc.

F ever

I nflammation

R educes TIAs due to fibrin platelet embolus

E liminates (reduces) death with hx of MI

Annie (git yer gun) Aspirin is busy "firing" at platelets to reduce the blood coagulation in her body, especially with myocardial infarction or transient ischemic attack. She is holding her stomach as this med can cause stomach irritation. "FIRE" reviews other indications for prescribing aspirin.

GLYCOPROTEIN IIB/IIIA INHIBITORS

Action: Antiplatelet action. Platelet glycoprotein antagonist. This agent reversibly prevents fibrinogen, von Willebrand's factor from binding to the glycoprotein IIb/IIIa receptor, inhibiting platelett aggregation.

Indications: Acute coronary syndrome including those with PCI (percutaneous coronary intervention)

Warnings: **HIGH ALERT DRUG** Hypersensitivity, active internal bleeding; history of bleeding. CVA within 1 month. Major surgery with severe trauma, severe hypotension, history of intracranial bleeding, intracranial neoplasm, arteriovenous malformation/aneurysm, aortic dissection, dependence on renal dialysis. Severe uncontrolled hypertension.

Other Specific Information: Increased bleeding with aspirin, heparin, NSAIDs, anticoagulants, ticlopidine, clopidogrel, dipyridamole, thrombolytics, plicamycin, valproate, abciximab. Do not administer with platelet receptor inhibitors IIb, IIIa.

Interventions: Assess platelets, Hgb, Hct, creatinine, PT/APTT baseline INR within 6 hr of loading dose and qd thereafter. Clients undergoing PCI should have ACT evaluated; the APTT should be between 50–70 sec. unless PCI is to be performed; during PCI, ACT should be 300–350 sec; if platelets drop<100,000/mm3, review additional platelet count; discontinue drug if thrombocytopenia is confirmed and also draw a Hct, Hgb, and serum creatinine. Assess for bleeding (i.e., gums, bruising, petechiae, ecchymosis; GI, GU tract, cardiac cath sites, or IM injection sites). Aspirin and heparin may be given with this drug. D/C heparin prior to removing any femoral artery sheaths after PCI. Do not administer discolored solutions or those with particulates, discard unused amount. Discontinue drug prior to CABG.

Education: Review reason for taking the medication. Instruct the importance of reporting bruising, bleeding and chest pain. Half-life is 2.5 hr, steady state 4–6 hr, metabolism limited, excretion via kidneys. Creatinine clearance will be calculated prior to starting medication.

Evaluation: Client will experience therapeutic effects from the medication with no undesirable effects.

Drugs: eptifibatide (Integrilin), Aggrestate, Reopro

EPTIFIBATIDE (INTEGRILIN)

HIGH ALERT

S urgery—previous 6 weeks

P lanned administration of parenteral GP II b/IIIa

R enal dialysis

U ncontrolled hypertension

C VA within 30 days of hemorrhagic CVA

E vidence of a bleeding disorder
   valuate creatinine clearance

If serum creatinine more than 2 mg/dl or estimated CrCl less than 50 mL/min., reduce continuous infusion rate to 1 mcg/Kg/min.

To estimate CrCl, use the following formula
(calulation to be verified by two people)

$$CrCl - \frac{(140 - age)(Weight\ in\ Kg)}{72\ (serum\ creatinine)}$$
Multiply by 0.85 if female

CrCl = _____ mL/min

©2005 I CAN Publishing, Inc.

Remember, the "SPRUCE" tree is falling down. If "SPRUCE" is present, do not administer Integrilin.

CLOPIDOGREL
(PLAVIX)

Action: Platelet aggregation inhibitor by inhibiting the first and second phases of ADP-induced effects in platelet aggregation.

Indications: Reduces atherosclerotic events such as a stroke, MI, vascular death, or peripheral vascular disease

Warnings: Hypersensitivity, pathologic bleeding (i.e., peptic ulcers, intracranial hemorrhage), lactation

Undesirable Effects: Depression, dizziness, fatigue, headache, epistaxis, cough, chest pain, hypertension, GI BLEEDING, abdominal pain, diarrhea, dyspepsia, gastritis, pruritus, purpura, rash, BLEEDING, NEUTROPEINA, THROMBOCYTOPENIC PURPURA, hypercholesterolemia, arthralgia, back pain, Hypersensitivity reactions including ANGIOEDEMA, ANAPHYLACTOID REACTIONS, BRONCHOSPASM

Other Specific Information: Concurrent abciximab, eptifibatide, tirofiban, aspirin, NSAIDs, heparin, heparinoids, thrombolytic agents, ticlopidine, or warfarin may increase bleeding. Plavix may decrease metabolism and increase effects of phenytoin, tolbutamide, tamoxifen, torsemide, fluvastatin, warfarin, and many NSAIDs.

Interventions: Assess for symptoms of stroke, MI during treatment. Liver function studies: AST, ALT, bilirubin, creatinine (long -term therapy). Blood studies: CBC, Hct, Hgb, PT, cholesterol (long-term therapy)

Education: Educate client that blood work will be necessary during treatment. Report any unusual bruising or bleeding. Recommend taking with food or just after eating to minimize GI discomfort. Report diarrhea, skin rashes, chills, fever, sore throat, or subcutaneous bleeding. All health care providers must be told that clopidogrel is being used.

Staff Education: Do not confuse Plavix with Paxil or Elavil.

Evaluation: Client will not experience any occurrence of atherosclerotic events.

Drugs: clopidogrel (Plavix)

PLAVIX

B leeding, bronchospasms—undesirable effects

L owers risk of atherosclerotic events

E valuate bruising

E valuate liver function and blood studies

D rug/drug interactions are many!

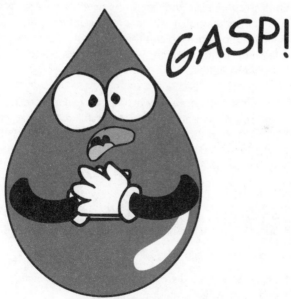

GASP!

©2005 I CAN Publishing, Inc.

"BLEED" will help you remember some important facts regarding Plavix.

THROMBOLYTIC AGENTS

Action: Binds with plasminogen causing conversion to plasmin, which dissolves blood clots.

Indications: Dissolves blood clots due to coronary artery thrombi, deep vien thrombosis, pulmonary embolism.

Warnings: Active internal bleeding; recent CVA; aneurysm; hypertension; anticoagulant therapy; ulcerative colitis. Severe allergic reactions to either anistreplase or streptokinase. Caution: Alphabet Soup names = high error risk. TNK is weight-based. TPA is the only thrombolytic approved for use in non-hemorrhagic stroke.

Undesirable Effects: Hemorrhage, headache, nausea, rash, fever, bleeding, allergic reaction, hypotension.

Other Specific Information: Client's risk of bleeding is increased. Aminocaproic acid inhibits streptokinase and cannot be used to reverse its fibri-nolytic effects. Effects of drug disappear within a few hours after discontinuing, but the systemic effect of coagulation and the risk of bleeding may persist for 24 hours. Increase in risk for bleeding with heparin, oral anticoagulants, antiplatelet drugs, and NASIDs.

Interventions: Monitor CBC especially hgb/hct, coagulation tests. Evaluate bleeding at a sutured wound, arterial site, central line. Monitor vital signs during and after infusion; monitor EKG for re-perfusion dysrhythmias. Watch for unusual bleeding disturbance (GI, GU); initiate bleeding protocol measures for several hours (e.g., no venipunctures, repetitive manual blood pressure, or removal of IV lines or catheters).

Education: Explain the treatment to client and family. Explain need for frequent VS and other assessments. Instruct client to report any undesirable effects.

Evaluation: The client's clot has dissolved and there are no signs and symptoms of active bleeding or other undesirable effects.

Drugs: alteplase (Activase, tPA); anistreplace (APSAC, Eminase); streptokinase (Streptase); urokinase (Abbokinase); reteplase (rRA); tenecteplase (TNK)

ADAM ASE

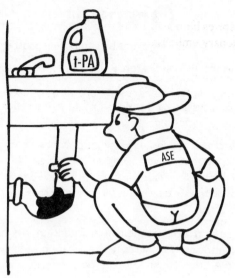

©2001 I CAN Publishing, Inc.

C BC, hgb, hct—monitor

L ook for dysrhythmias

O bserve for bleeding

T he vital signs must be monitored

    Adam **"ASE"** will dissolve the clog in this sink just as he dissolves the "CLOT" in a blood vessel. He will use t-PA or another thrombolytic agent that ends in **"ASE"**.

HEMORRHEOLOGIC AGENT: PENTOXIFYLLINE
(Trental)

Action: Blood viscosity reducing agent by stimulating prostacyclin formation.

Indications: Intermittent claudicaton. Related to chronic occlusive vascular disease.

Warnings: Hypersensitivity to this drug or xanthines; retinal/cerebral hemorrhage.

Undesirable Effects: Epistaxis, flu like symptoms, nasal congestion, laryngitis, leukopenia, malaise, weight changes, agitation, drowsiness, dizziness, nervous, insomnia, blurred vision, dyspnea, angina, arrhythmias, edema, flushing, hypotension, abdominal discomfort, belching, bloating, diarrhea, dyspepsia, flatus, nausea, vomiting, tremor.

Other Specific Information: Additive hypotension may occur with antihypertensives and nitrates. May increase the risk of bleeding with warfarin, heparin, aspirin, NSAIDs, cefamandole, cefoperazone, cefotetan, plicamycin, valproic acid, clopigogrel, ticlopidine, eptifibatide, tirofiban, or other thrombolytic agents. May increase the risk of theophylline toxicity.

Interventions: Assess blood pressure, respirations of client. If GI and CNS undesirable effects occur, decrease dose to twice daily; discontinue if effects continue. May cause dizziness and blurred vision; caution client to avoid driving and other activities requiring alertness until response to medication is determined. Administer with meals to prevent GI upset. Do not break, crush, or chew ext. released tabs.

Education: Advise client to avoid smoking due to nicotine constricting blood vessels. Instruct client to notify provider of care if nausea, vomiting, GI upset, drowsiness, dizziness, or headache persists. Advise client that it may take 2–4 weeks to maintain a therapeutic response. Decreased fats and cholesterol, increased exercise, decreased smoking are necessary to correct condition. Observe feet for arterial insufficiency. Use cotton socks, well-fitted shoes; not to go barefoot. Observe for bleeding, bruises, epistaxis. Avoid smoking to prevent blood vessel constriction.

Evaluation: Client will experience a decrease in pain and cramping and will have an increase in the ability to ambulate.

Drug: pentoxifylline (Trental)

TRENTAL

T aken 1x daily

R educes RBC aggregation and hyperviscosity

H **E** lps with signs and symptoms of Intermittent Claudication

N on-labeled FDA use for diabetic complications, acute alcoholic hepatitis

T oxic drug/drug effects with theophylline and other "xanthines"

A lways ask about recent surgeries, recent bleeding even retinal or cerebral

L ike client to take with meals or food

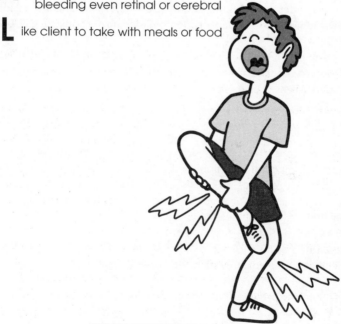

©2005 I CAN Publishing, Inc.

TRENT will be **ALL** better when his intermittent claudication subsides. The medication TRENTAL is used to decrease this medical condition.

BILE ACID SEQUESTRANT

Action: Combines with bile acids in the intestine resulting in excretion in the feces. Cholesterol is oxidized in the liver to replace the lost bile acids; serum cholesterol and LDL are decreased.

Indications: Hypercholesterolemia when dietary management does not lower cholesterol.

Warnings: Complete biliary obstruction, abnormal function of the intestine; hepatic or renal dysfunction; pregnancy, lactation; elderly client.

Undesirable Effects: Constipation, indigestion, nausea, vomiting, or GI bleeding; headache, syncope; increased bleeding tendencies due to vitamin K malabsorption; rash; muscle pain.

Other Specific Information: ↓ absorption of warfarin. ↓ absorption of digoxin, thiazides, propranolol, penicillin, tetracyclines, vancomycin, folic acid, and thyroid hormones. ↓ absorption of fat soluble vitamins (A, D, E, K).

Interventions: Monitor serum cholesterol, triacylglycerol levels, and PT in relation to baseline at regular intervals. Monitor appropriate drug levels based on current drug intake. Monitor I & O and bowel status.

Education: Take other meds 1 hour before or 4 to 6 hours after cholestyramines or colestipol. Diet low in fats, cholesterol, and sugars; high in fiber. Follow directions in mixing; never take as a dry powder. (Incomplete mixing may result in mucosal irritation!) Mix with 3–6 oz. water, milk, fruit juice, or soup. Take before meals and drink several glasses of water between meals. Instruct that a laxative or stool softener may assist in preventing constipation. Report unusual bleeding or bruising.

Evaluation: Serum cholesterol and low-density lipoprotein (LDL) levels will decrease and remain within the normal range.

Drugs: cholestyramine (Questran); colestipol (Colestid)

BILE-ACID SEQUESTRANT

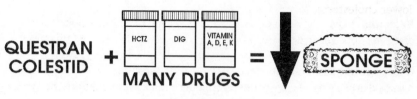

QUESTRAN
COLESTID
+

HCTZ   DIG   VITAMIN A, D, E, K

MANY DRUGS
=
SPONGE

©2001 I CAN PUBLISHING, INC.

L DL is ↓15–30%

I ncrease fluids and fiber

P T monitoring

I ncrease in GI distress—constipation

D ecreases absorption of many meds

FIBRIC ACID

Action: Increases activity of lipoprotein lipase, promoting VLDL and triacylglycerols catabolism. Promotes transfer of cholesterol to HDL. The reduction of triacylglycerols is significant.

Indications: Hyperlipidemia.

Warnings: Liver or renal disease, primary biliary cirrhosis, gallbladder disease, peptic ulcer disease.

Undesirable Effects: GI effects include abdominal distention, constipation, diarrhea, flatulence, nausea, vomiting; cholelithiasis; myositis; headache, dizziness, blurred vision with gemfibrozil; rash, urticaria; neutropenia, leuko-penia, anemia, or agranulocytosis.

Other Specific Information: May ↑ effect of warfarin, sulfonyureas, and insulin. Concomitant use of probenecid ↑ clofibrate levels. If gemfibrozil is administered with lovastatin, an ↑ risk of rhabdomyolysis and myoglobinuria may result in acute renal failure.

Interventions: Monitor liver/renal function tests, cholesterol, and tria-cylglycerol levels in relation to baseline and at regular intervals. Monitor serum glucose (if on antidiabetics), uric acid, and CBC. Monitor PT if client is taking oral anticoagulants. Monitor GI response and urine output.

Education: Attempt dietary corrections before meds. Encourage a diet low in fats, cholesterol, and/or sugars. Restrict alcohol. Instruct to take med before meals. Encourage weight reduction and physical exercise. Instruct that a paradoxic rise in levels may occur in the initial 2 or 3 months, but decrease after this period. Instruct regarding the importance of keeping clinical appointments for laboratory studies and reevaluation by the provider.

Evaluation: Serum cholesterol and triacylglycerol levels will be reduced to normal limits.

Drugs: clofibrate (Atromid-S); gemfibrozil (Lopid)

FIBRIC ACID

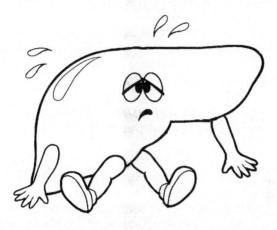

L iver or renal disease—WARNING

I ncreases effect of warfarin or sulfonlyureas

V LDL, LDL, triacylglycerols and cholesterol—monitor

E ncourage diet ↓ in fat, cholesterol and sugars

R estrict alcohol

HMG CoA INHIBITORS

Action: The "statins" are competitive inhibitors of HMG-CoA reductase, an enzyme necessary for cholesterol biosynthesis in the intestine and liver.

Indications: Hypercholesterolemia; ↓ low-density lipoprotein (LDL); ↑ high-density lipoprotein (HDL).

Warnings: Active liver disease; unexplained, persistent elevations in liver function tests. Caution: alcoholism; acute infections; metabolic disorders; electrolyte imbalance; hypotension.

Undesirable Effects: GI distress: (dyspepsia, diarrhea, constipation, gas); headache; blurred vision with lovastatin. Rare: liver dysfunction, myalgia, myopathy, or myositis.

Other Specific Information: ↑ effect of warfarin. Bile acid binding acids may ↓ availability of "statin". Digoxin ↑ "statin" levels. Concomitant use of ACE inhibitors may result in ↑ K+. Concomitant use of erythromycin, fibric acid derivatives, immunosuppressive drugs, and niacin may ↑ rhabdomyolysis.

Interventions: Monitor serum cholesterol and triacylglycerol levels, serum creatine kinase (CK), and LFT in relation to baseline and at regular intervals. Discontinue "statins" if LFT ↑ > 3 times normal. Prior to initiating drug therapy, encourage appropriate diet, exercise, and weight reduction.

Education: Drink 2–3 liters of fluid daily. Take with food and at bedtime; reduce cholesterol, fats, and sugar; diet high in fiber (whole grain cereals, fruits, and vegetables). Exercise and weight reduction should also be encouraged for obese clients along with therapy. It may take several weeks before blood lipid levels decrease. If taking lovastatin, report changes in vision and have an annual eye exam.

Evaluation: Serum cholesterol and triacylglycerol levels will decrease and return to the normal limits. The HDL serum level will have a modest increase.

Drugs: (*These drugs end in "statin".*) atorva**statin** (Lipitor); ceriva**statin** (Baycol); fluva**statin** (Lescol); lova**statin** (Mevacor); prava**statin** (Pravachol); simva**statin** (Zocor)

L. L. STATIN

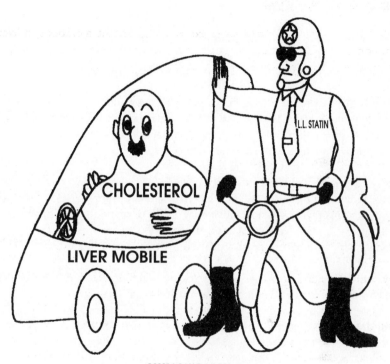

CHOLESTEROL

LIVER MOBILE

L.L. STATIN

©2001 I CAN Publishing, Inc.

Officer "L. L. (lipid lowering) Statin" has stopped the liver mobile and its driver, Cholesterol. These drugs lower cholesterol and can be highly toxic to the liver. Drugs that are in this group end in **"statin"**.

NIACIN

Action: Inhibits free fatty acid release from adipose tissue by inhibiting accumulation of cAMP stimulated by lipolytic hormones. Increases rate of triacylglycerol removal from the plasma.

Indication: Hyperlipidemia.

Warnings: Acute MI, heart failure; diabetes mellitus; gout; hepatic/renal dysfunction; active peptic ulcer disease; concomitant HMG-CoA reductase inhibitors; severe hypotension; arterial hemorrhage; pregnancy.

Undesirable Effects: Headache, GI upset, flushing and itching over upper body (face, neck, arms) with raised rash appearance (resolves approximately $1/2$–1 hour after ingestion), hyperglycemia, hyperuricemia, myalgia, cardiac dysrhythmias in those with coronary artery disease.

Other Specific Information: Most severe cases of hepatotoxicity have been reported with SR forms. Flushing is ↓ with SR preps, but GI effects are ↑. Lovastatin, pravastatin, simvastatin may ↑ risk of rhabdomyolysis and acute renal failure. ↑ effectiveness of antihypertensives, vasoactive drugs. ↑ risk of bleeding with anticoagulants. ↓ absorption with bile acid sequestrants.

Interventions: Monitor liver function tests, serum uric acid, serum glucose, and cholesterol in relation to baseline and at regular intervals. Monitor PT and platelets if taking an anticoagulant. Monitor for flushing, discomfort after medicating (i.e., headache, dizziness, blurred vision), or orthostatic hypotension.

Education: Take with food and at bedtime. Avoid alcohol and take bile acid sequestrant (if prescribed) 4–6 hours apart. Pretreatment with 325 mg ASA may ↓ undesirable effect of vasodilation. Follow diet regimen-low cholesterol and low saturated fats. If dizziness occurs, change position slowly. Undesirable effects are typically transient and will usually subside with continued therapy. Review importance for follow-up evaluation during long-term therapy.

Evaluation: LDL and triacylglycerol levels will decrease and return to normal limits. HDL will increase.

Drug: niacin (Niaspan)

NIACIN

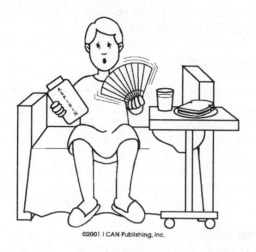

©2001 I CAN Publishing, Inc.

N ote liver function tests—regular intervals

I tching and flushing—U E

A spirin before Niacin may ↓ U E of vasodilation

C ontraindications: hepatic disease, pregnancy

I nstruct to take with food and at bedtime

N o high cholesterol foods

ANTILIPEMIC: ZETIA

Action: Inhibits absorption of cholesterol by the small intestine.

Indications: Hypercholesterolemia, homozygous familial hypercholesterolemia, homozygous sitosterolemia.

Warnings: Hypersensitivity, severe hepatic disease.

Undesirable Effects: Fatigue, dizziness. Nausea, diarrhea, abdominal pain. Chest pain. Myalgias, arthralgias, back pain. Pharyngitis, sinusitis, cough.

Other Specific Information: Toxicity: cyclosporine. Decreased action of ezetimibe with antacids, cholestyramine.
Increased action of ezetimibe with fibric acid derivatives.

Interventions: Assess lipid levels, LFTs baseline and periodically during treatment. Administer without regard to meals.

Education: Advise the importance for compliance. Review the importance of decreasing risk factors: high-fat diet, smoking, alcohol consumption, absence of exercise. Notify provider if suspect pregnancy.

Evaluation: Decrease in the cholesterol.

Drug: ezetimibe (Zetia)

ZETIA

Di Z zines, respiratory, HA, diarrhea may
be side effects

E ncourage use of contraceptive barriers if
used with "STATINS"

T aken without regard to food

I nhibits absorption of dietary cholesterol

A djunct to diet & exercise

©2005 I CAN Publishing, Inc.

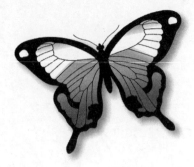

Do not think that the knowledge you presently possess is changeless, absolute truth. Avoid being narrow- minded and bound to present views. Learn and practice non-attachment from view in order to be open to receive others' veiwpoints. Truth is found in life and not merely in conceptual knowledge. Be ready to learn throughout your entire life and to observe reality in yourself and in the world at all times.

Thich Nhat Hanh

Respiratory
Agents

CONCEPT: BRONCHODILATORS

Breathing and coughing techniques: This will facilitate the removal of respiratory secretions and optimize oxygen exchange.

Relaxation techniques: Since anxiety may result in respiratory difficulty, review ways to alleviate anxiety such as music and relaxation techniques.

Evaluate heart rate and BP: Teach client to monitor heart rate and BP since an undesirable effect of these medications may be tachycardia, cardiac arrhythmias, and a change in blood pressure. (Beta$_2$ Adrenergic Agonists can cause hypertension; methylxanthines can cause hypotension at theophylline levels > 30-35 mcg/ml.)

Arm identification: Recommend clients having asthmatic attacks to wear an ID bracelet or tag.

Tremors: Evaluate client for tremors from these medications.

Have 8 or more glasses of fluids: Fluid will assist in decreasing the viscosity of the respiratory secretions.

Emphasize no smoking: Encourage the client to stop smoking under medical supervision.

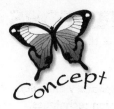
Concept

BRONCHODILATORS

B reathing and coughing techniques

R elaxation techniques

E valuate heart rate and blood pressure

A rm identification

T remors

H ave 8 or more glasses of fluids

E mphasize no smoking

©2001 I CAN Publishing, Inc.

ANTIHISTAMINES

Action: Blocks histamine release at H_1 receptors.

Indications: Upper respiratory allergic disorders; anaphylactic reactions; blood transfusion reactions; acute urticaria; motion sickness.

Warnings: Allergies, acute asthmatic attack, lower respiratory disease, hepatic disorder, narrow-angle glaucoma, symptomatic prostatic hypertrophy, pregnancy, lactation.

Undesirable Effects: Depression, sedation, dry mouth, GI upset, bronchospasm, thickening of secretions, (anticholinergic effects), arrhythmias.

Other Specific Information: Alcohol, CNS depressants may ↑ CNS depressant effect. Ketoconazole may alter metabolism of antihistamine. ↑ levels and possible toxicity with ketoconazole, erythromycin when given with fexofenadine. Avoid MAO inhibitors

Interventions: Monitor vital signs, intake and output. If secretions are thick, use a humidifier.

Education: Instruct client to take with food; drink a minimum of 8 glasses of fluid per day. Advise to do frequent mouth care; may use sugarless gum, lozenges, or candy. Notify provider if confusion or other undesirable effects occur. Instruct client not to drive or operate machinery if drowsiness occurs or until response to drug has been determined. For prophylaxis of motion sickness, recommend taking 30–60 minutes before traveling. Avoid alcohol and other CNS depressants.

Evaluation: Client will have improvement of histamine-associated (*i.e., rhinitis, conjunctivitis, motion sickness, etc.*) with no undesirable effects from the medication.

Drugs: azatadine (Optimine); azelastine (Astelin); brompheniramine (Dimetapp); buclizine (Bucladin-S); cetirizine (Zyrtec); chlorpheniramine (Chlor-Trimeton); clemastine (Tavist); cyclizine (Mazerine); cyproheptadine (Periactin); dexchlorpheniramine (Polaramine); dimenhydrinate (Dramamine); diphenhydramine (Benadryl); fexofenadine (Allegra); hydroxyzine (Atarax, Vistaril); loratidine (Claritin); meclizine (Antivert); promethazine (Phenergan); tripelennamine (PBZ)

ANTIHISTAMINES

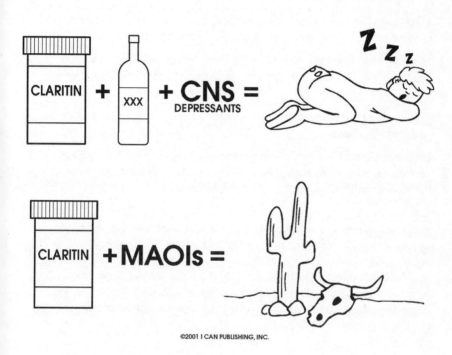

©2001 I CAN PUBLISHING, INC.

Antihistamines (Claritin) combined with alcohol and CNS depressant may result in sleep. Antihistamines and MAOIs may result in dryness.

BETA$_2$ ADRENERGIC AGONISTS

Action: Stimulates beta receptors in lung. Relaxes bronchial smooth muscle. Increases vital capacity; decreases airway resistance.

Indications: Asthma, bronchitis, emphysema, relief of bronchospasm occurring during anesthesia, exercised-induced bronchospasm.

Warnings: Hypersensitivity, angina, tachycardia, cardiac arrhythmias, hypertension, cardiac disease, narrow-angle glaucoma, hepatic disease.

Undesirable Effects: Nervousness, tremors, restlessness, insomnia, headache; nausea, vomiting; tachycardia, irregular heart beat, hypertension, cardiac dysrhythmia.

Other Specific Information: ↑ effects with other sympathomimetics. ↓ with beta blockers.

Interventions: Monitor breath sounds; sensorium levels for confusion and restlessness due to hypoxia; and vital signs (pulse and blood pressure can increase greatly). Check for cardiac dysrhythmias.

Education: Caution against overuse. Notify provider before taking other meds or if symptoms are not relieved. Demonstrate correct use of inhalers or nebulizers. Teach about metered-dose inhalers (MDI). When two puffs are needed, 1–3 minutes should lapse between the two puffs. A spacer may be used to increase the delivery of the medication. If a glucocorticoid inhalant is to be used with a bronchodilator, wait 5–15 minutes before using the inhaler containing the steroid for the bronchodilator effect. Assist client in identifying the cause of the acute bronchial attack. (Refer to **"BREATHE"**.)

Evaluation: Client will be able to breathe without wheezing and without undesirable effects of the drug. Client will be able to participate in activities of daily living without dyspnea.

Drugs: (*Nonselective Adrenergic*): epinephrine (Adrenalin); (*Nonselective Beta-Adrenergic*): isoproterenol (Isuprel); (*Selective B$_2$*): albuterol (Proventil, Ventolin); bitolterol (Tornalate); isoetharine (Bronkosol); metaproterenol (Alupent); pirbuterol (Maxair); salmeterol (Serevent); terbutaline (Brethine, Bricanyl)

MAX AIR

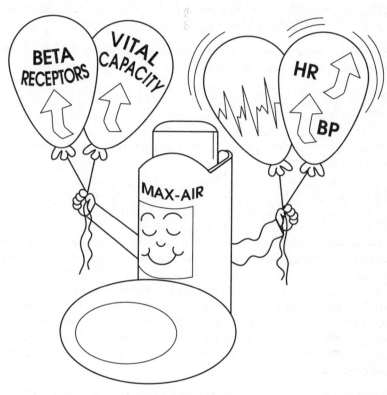

©2001 I CAN Publishing, Inc.

Max Air is smiling because he has been able to relieve bronchospasms from asthma and other respiratory diseases. He has plenty of air to breathe and blow up the balloons in the right hand. His left hand is shaky and weak. His heart is beating fast and his blood pressure is up from undesirable effects of his medication.

XANTHINES

Action: Inhibits phosphodiesterase, an enzyme responsible for breaking down cyclic AMP, resulting in bronchodilation and reducing airway resistance.

Indications: Asthma, emphysema, chronic obstructive pulmonary disease (COPD), or chronic airway limitations (CAL).

Warnings: Uncontrolled seizure disorder, cardiovascular disorder, peptic ulcer disease, young children and elderly.

Undesirable Effects: Uncommon at serum levels below 20mcg/ml; levels > 20mcg/ml—nausea (first sign of toxicity), vomiting, headache, dizziness, insomnia, irritability; levels > 35mcg/ml—tremors (later sign of toxicity), nervousness, tachycardia, palpitations, hypotension, cardicac dysrhythmias, seizures, death.

Other Specific Information: Cimetidine, oral contraceptives, and several antibiotics (ciproflaxacin, norflaxacin, erythomycin) ↑ toxicity. ↓ effects of neuromuscular blockers, phenytoin, and lithium. ↓ effect with smoking, rifampin, phenobarbital, corticosteroids, and others. Charcoal-broiled food, high-protein, low carbohydrate diet may increase theophylline elimination.

Interventions: Monitor ABG's and theophylline levels (normal level is 10-20 mcg/ml). Peak serum concentration should be taken 1 hour after I.V., 1-2 hours following immediate-release dose, 3-8 hours following extended release. Take trough level just before next dose. Take oral preparation 1 hr. before or 2 hrs. after meals. Monitor vital signs, respirations, and breath sounds.

Education: Instruct to avoid use of caffeine derivatives (chocolate, coffee, tea, cola, cocoa). Caution not to take OTC meds that contain ephedrine or sympathomimetics. (Refer to "**BREATHE**".)

Evaluation: Client will be able to breathe without wheezing. Serum theophylline levels will be in the normal range.

Drugs: aminophylline (theophylline ethylenediamine); theophylline Immediate-release: (Aerolate, Slo-Phyllin, Theolair,) Extended-release: (Slo-Bid, Theo-Dur, Theo-24, Uni-Dur Uniphyl)

AMILY TOXICITY

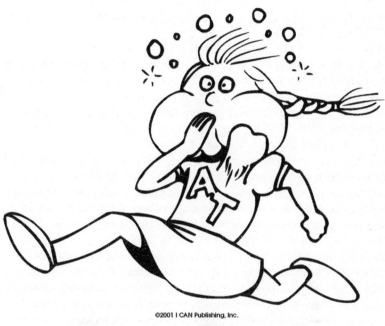

©2001 I CAN Publishing, Inc.

Amily Toxicity

Amily represents some of the most commonly occurring undesirable effects: nausea (first sign of toxicity), arrhythmias, tachyacardia, nervousness (jumpimg up) and tremors (later sign of toxicity).

CORTICOSTEROID INHALERS

Action: Decreases inflammation and edema in respiratory tract. Reduces bronchoconstriction and secretion of mucus.

Indications: Chronic asthma; exacerbation of COPD or CAL.

Warnings: Bronchiectasis; Systemic fungal infections; persistently positive sputum culture for candida albicans. *Caution:* adrenal insufficiency; pregnancy/lactation.

Undesirable Effects: Usually does not induce systemic toxicity. Risk of oral candida albicans infection (thrush). Sore throat, an unpleasant taste in mouth, or dysphonia may occur.

Other Specific Information: Mild suppression of the pituitary-adrenal axis may occur with prolonged use. Decreased steroid levels with barbiturates, phenytoin, rifampin. Decreased effectiveness of salicylates.

Interventions: Monitor respiratory status on an ongoing basis.

Education: Instruct not to use for acute attacks. If taking bronchodilators, instruct client to use bronchodilator before corticosteroid aerosol. After inhaling, the client should hold the inhaled drug for a few seconds before exhaling. Allow 1–3 minutes to elapse between each inhalation. Rinse mouth with water after inhalations. A spacer is particularly important for client inhaling corticosteroids. It will reduce risk of steroid-associated oropharyngeal candidiasis. Keep inhaler clean and unobstructed. Wash in warm water and dry thoroughly. Notify provider if sore throat or sore mouth occurs; do not stop abruptly. Must taper off gradually under provider supervision. Encourage the use of a diary to record administration of meds and the clinical response.

Evaluation: The client will experience fewer asthmatic episodes of lesser severity without undesirable effects.

Drugs: beclomethasone (Beclovent, Vanceril); flunisolide (AeroBid, AeroBid-M); triamcinolone (Azmacort)

ASTHMA

A ction = decreased respiratory track edema

S pacer use recommended

T hrush

H ave client use bronchodilator first

M ust taper off gradually

A sthma control—not acute attacks

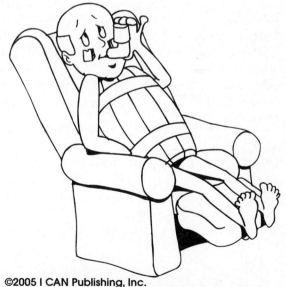

©2005 I CAN Publishing, Inc.

LEUKOTRIENE RECEPTOR ANTAGONIST

Action: Blocks the receptor that inhibits leukotriene formation, preventing many of the signs of asthma.

Indications: Prophylaxis and chronic treatment of asthma in adults and children > 6yrs. old.

Warnings: Hypersensitivity; acute asthmatic attacks; pregnancy/lactation.

Undesirable Effects: Headache, dizziness; nausea, diarrhea; nasal congestion. More serious undesirable effects can occur if client is taking zafirlukast (i.e., *Churg-Strauss syndrome, which presents with eosinophilia, vasculitic rash, cardiac and pulmonary complications*) when oral steroid dose is decreased.

Other Specific Information: ↓ effects if taking montelukast with phenobarbital, rifampin. Numerous interactions may occur when taking zafirlukast. Propranolol, theophylline, and warfarin levels may have ↑ effects when given with zileuton.

Intereventions: Monitor breath sounds and for gastric distress. Monitor liver function tests when client is taking zieleuton.

Education: Recommend taking drug in the evening without regard to food. Not effective for acute asthma attack or acute bronchospasm. Instruct regarding the importance of avoiding aspirin or NSAIDs in clients with hypersensitivities while they are taking this drug. Review the importance of having alternative medication available for an acute asthma attack. Review safety precautions if dizziness occurs.

Evaluation: Client will be free from signs and symptoms of asthma.

Drugs: montelukast (Singulair); zafirlukast (Accolate); zileuton (Zyflo)

LOOK! A TRAIN!

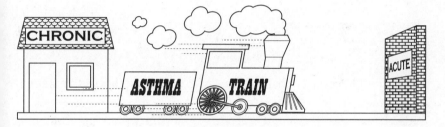

©2001 I CAN Publishing, Inc.

It is OK to board the train in the town of Chronic, but it is too late by the time the train gets to the town of Acute (asthma).

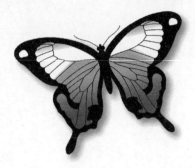

The Universe is change; our life is what our thoughts make it.

Marcus Aurelius Antoninus

Love is, above all else, the gift of oneself.

Jean Anouth

Anti-Infective
Agents

CONCEPT: ANTIBIOTICS

Monitor superinfections: Monitor for a secondary infection (bacterial or fungal growth) due to drug therapy. Assess for signs and symptoms of stomatitis (mouth ulcers), furry black tongue; genital discharge (vaginitis); and anal or genital itching. Elderly clients, children, and clients with a depressed immune system should be monitored carefully.

Evaluate renal/liver functions: Since many antibiotics are metabolized in the liver and excreted via the kidneys, it is of paramount importance to have adequate functioning of these two systems. Evaluate laboratory tests for liver and kidney function; these include liver enzymes, BUN, and serum creatinine.

Diarrhea: Recommend that client eat yogurt to prevent this undesirable effect.

Inform provider prior to taking other meds: Due to the possibility of drug-drug interactions it important that the client understands the reason to discuss this with the provider. It is also important to evaluate the current medications the client is taking for potential interactions.

Cultures prior to initial dose: Prior to the initial dose, obtain and send blood cultures to the laboratory to identify the organism and antibiotic sensitivity.

Alcohol is out; ask about allergy: Instruct client to drink no alcohol. If there has been a previous problem with an allergic reaction, do not administer the medicine. The most serious allergic reaction is anaphylaxis. It begins with diffuse flushing, itching, and a general warm feeling. Hives may be present on the client's face, neck, and chest. As this progresses, generalized edema develops. As the face becomes involved, there is a concern with upper airway edema, with potential respiratory difficulty and impending obstruction. This may result in respiratory wheezing, stridor, and shortness of breath.

Take full course of pills: An ineffective course of antibiotics will allow the bacteria to mutate and develop resistance to the antibiotic. It is important that the medicines are not shared with friends and family due to the risk of allergies and may not be appropriate for the specific bacterial growth. Review the importance of not taking medicines that have been in the cabinet for a while since some medicines may become toxic as they degenerate past the date of expiration.

Evaluate cultures, WBC, temperature, blood dyscrasias, and serum electrolytes: A positive response to the therapy is evaluated by negative cultures, WBCs and body temperature within normal range. Since some antibiotics such as penicillin can cause neutropenia or thrombocytopenia, clients must be monitored for blood dyscrasias. The undesirable effect of diarrhea may result in hypokalemia. Hypernatremia may also occur in clients receiving prolonged treatment with intravenous antibiotics.

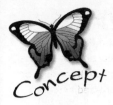
Concept

ANTIBIOTICS

M onitor superinfections

E valuate renal/liver functions

D iarrhea—take yogurt

I nform provider prior to taking other meds

C ultures prior to initial dose

A lcohol is out, ask about allergy

T ake full course (of pills)

E valuate cultures, WBC, temperature, blood

©2001 I CAN Publishing, Inc.

AMINOGLYCOSIDES

Action: Bactericidal. Binds with 30s or 50s ribosomal subunit, thus inhibiting protein synthesis.

Indications: Serious infections caused by gram-negative infections (*ie., Enterobacter, Escherichia coli, Klebsiella, Proteus, Pseudomonas, and Serratia*). Streptomycin is one of the drugs primarily used for tuberculosis.

Warnings: Hypersensitivity; renal impairment; vestibular/cochlear impairment; decreased neuromuscular transmission (*i.e., myasthenia gravis, Parkinson's disease*); heart failure; elderly.

Undesirable Effects: Anorexia, nausea, tremors, tinnitus, photosensitivity, superinfection, or agranulocytosis. Significant potential for neurotoxicity, nephrotoxicity, and ototoxicity with high levels for extended periods. Aminoglycoside nephrotoxicity is usually seen as a gradual increase in creatinine over several days. Acute, large changes in creatinine should be investigated for other causes.

Other Specific Information: Loop diuretics may ↑ ototoxic potential when given with this class. Penicillins, vancomycin, amphotericin B, and furosemide may ↑ nephrotoxicity.

Interventions: BUN/creatinine, audiograms, and vestibular function studies should also be monitored periodically during an extended high dose therapy over 10 days. Adjust for renal insufficiency. Monitor vital signs and peak and trough serum levels routinely. For IV administration, dilute and administer slowly over 60 minutes to prevent toxicity. Monitor I & O; hydrate well before and during therapy. If prescribed oral drug, take full course and drink plenty of fluids. If anorexia or nausea occurs, provide small, frequent meals. Establish plan for safety if vestibular nerve effects occur. (Refer to "**MEDICATE**".) Ensure levels are drawn per hospital policy.

Education: Administer other antibiotics 1 hour before/after oral aminoglycosides. Recommend using sun block and protective clothing when exposed to the sun. (Refer to "**MEDICATE**".)

Evaluation: Client's body temperature, WBC count, and cultures will return to normal range.

Drugs: amikacin (Amikin); gentamicin (Garamycin, Jenamicin); kanamycin (Kantrex, Klebcil); neomycin (Mycifradin, Neobiotic); streptomycin (Streptomycin); tobramycin (Nebcin)

AMINO MICE

Genta**myc**in
Amikacin
Kana**myc**in
Neo**myc**in
Strepto**myc**in
Tobra**myc**in

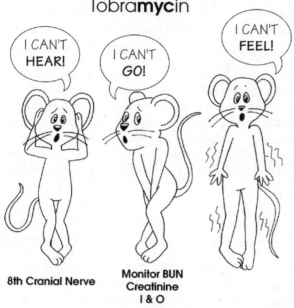

8th Cranial Nerve   Monitor BUN
                         Creatinine
                         I & O

©2001 I CAN Publishing, Inc.

Three Amino Mice
(sung to the tune of "Three Blind Mice")

One can't feel,	Vestibular function and audiograms
One can't hear.	Should always be studied in patient care plans
One can't pee—	*[or "as part of your plan"]*
They're toxic mice, all three.	Grab BUNs and creatinine as quick as you can,
	Yes! Three amino mice.

Our 3 "Amino Mice" will assist you in remembering 3 major undesirable effects of this category of drugs: "ototoxicity", "nephrotoxicity", and "neurotoxicity".

CEPHALOSPORINS

Action: Inhibits bacterial cell wall synthesis. Most effective against rapidly growing organisms.

Indications: 1st generation: Often used in clients allergic to penicillin. Gram-positive organisms and moderate activity against gram-negative organisms. **2nd generation:** Gram-negative organisms. **3rd generation:** Mostly gram-negative organisms. **4th generation:** Gram-negative and gram-positive organisms.

Warnings: Hypersensitivity to cephalosporins or penicillin. Caution with renal/hepatic impairment, bleeding disorders, or GI disease.

Undesirable Effects: Our friend the "**GIANT**" on the next page will help you remember these effects.

Other Specific Information: Cefamandole, cefmetazole, cefoperazone, or cefotetan may result in a disulfiram (Antabuse)–type reaction with alcohol consumption, or an ↑risk of bleeding when given with anticoagulants, or thrombolytic agents. The same drugs (with the exception of cefmetazole) when given with NSAIDs, especially aspirin, ↑ the risk of hemorrhaging. Probenecid may ↑ serum levels of cephalosporins resulting in potential toxicity.

Interventions: Monitor WBC counts, cultures, and PT. Assess BUN and creatinine levels in clients with renal impairment. Monitor VS, I & O, and undesirable effects. If client is a diabetic, monitor glucose levels. For IV administration, refer to drug circular for specific procedure. (Refer to "**MEDICATE**".)

Education: Administer on an empty stomach for better results. May take with food if gastric irritation develops. Use glucose-enzymatic tests such as Clinistix or Tes-Tape to decrease false-positive results. (Refer to "**MEDICATE**".)

Evaluation: Negative cultures. WBC count and body temperature will be within normal range.

Drugs: *First generation:* cefadroxil (Duricef); cefazolin (Ancef, Kefzol); cephalexin (Keflex); cephapirin (Cefadyl); cephradine (Velosef); *Second generation:* cefaclor (Ceclor); cefamandole (Mandol); cefditoren pivosil (Spectrcef); cefmetazole (Zefazone); cefonicid (Monocid); cefotetan (Cefotan); cefoxitin (Mefoxin); cefprozil (Cefzil); cefuroxime (Ceftin, Zinacef); loracarbef (Lorabid); *Third generation:* cefdinir (Omnicef); cefixime (Suprax); cefoperazone (Cefobid); cefotaxime (Claforan); cefpodoxime (Vantin); ceftazidime (Fortaz); ceftibuten (Cedax), ceftizoxime (Cefizox); ceftriaxone (Rocephin); *Fourth generation:* cefepime (Maxipime)

CEF THE GIANT

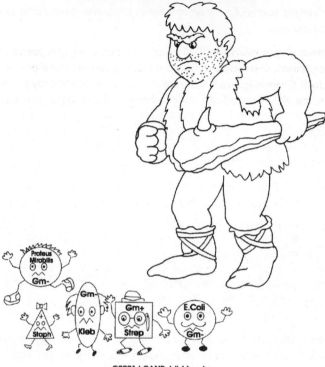

©2001 I CANPublishing, Inc.

GI: nausea, vomiting, diarrhea

Increase in glucose values

Anaphylaxis may occur; alcohol may cause vomiting

Nephrotoxicity

Thrombocytopenia

Cef/Ceph, the "GIANT" is a powerful antibiotic that can destroy several types of bacteria and represents the 1st generation of cephalosporins. He can also produce "GIANT" undesirable effects.

FLUOROQUINOLONES

Action: Bactericidal. Inhibits bacterial DNA synthesis via inhibition of DNA gyrase.

Indications: Broad spectrum. Wide range of susceptible gram-negative and gram-positive organisms. (*i.e., E. coli, P. Pseudomonas aeruginosa*). Used for urinary tract infections UTIs), bronchitis, sexually transmitted diseases, bone or joint, or ophthalmic infections. Individual fluoroquinolones vary in their spectrum of activity. All are indicated for UTIs, but only ciprofloxacin is approved for bone cancer and joint infections. (*It is beyond the scope of this book to review every individual drug indications. We refer you to current references.*)

Warnings: Hypersensitivity in children < 18 years of age. Children, pregnancy, lactation; hepatic or renal impairment; CNS disorders, or seizures.

Undesirable Effects: Hypersensitivity. Nausea, vomiting, diarrhea, headache, dizziness, photosensitivity. Rare effects include confusion, hallucinations, psychosis, and tremors.

Other Specific Information: Antacids, iron, sucralfate may ↓ absorption of drug up to 98%. May ↑ effects of theophylline and warfarin. ↑ risk of photosensitivity reactions with St. John's Wort therapy.

Interventions: Monitor temperature, WBC counts, cultures, symptoms of infection, BUN, and serum creatinine levels. Monitor I & O and vital signs. Maintain a urinary output of at least 1200 to 1500 ml daily. Slowly infuse IV ciprofloxacin and ofloxacin into a large vein over 1 hour to minimize vein irritation. Refer to drug circular for procedure. (Refer to "**MEDICATE**".)

Education: Instruct to take 2 hours after meals or 2 hours before or after antacids or iron. If GI distress occurs, take with food. Administer with full glass of water. Drink 6–8 glasses (8 oz.) of fluid daily. Protect against sunlight. Advise client to avoid hazardous activities that require alertness until the CNS response has been determined. (Refer to "**MEDICATE**".)

Evaluation: Negative cultures. Body temperature and WBC count within normal range.

Drugs: (*Many of these drugs end in "floxacin"*) cipro**floxacin** (Ciloxan, Cipro); enoxacin (Penetrex); gati**floxacin** (Tequin); levo**floxacin** (Levaquin); lome**floxacin** (Maxaquin); moxi**floxacin** (Avelox); nor**floxacin** (Noroxin); o**floxacin** (Floxin, Ocuflox); spar**floxacin** (Zagam); trova**floxacin** (Trovan)

T. T. FLOXACIN

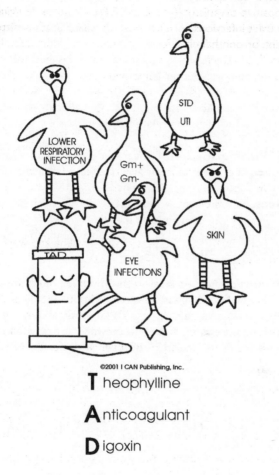

©2001 I CAN Publishing, Inc.

T heophylline

A nticoagulant

D igoxin

T.T. Floxacin and his flock are relieving themselves on TAD the fire hydrant. **T**heophylline, **A**nticoagulants, and **D**ig may result in drug toxicity when taken with the fluoroquinolones. This group of drugs ends in **floxacin** and is used to treat urinary tract infections as well as a wide range of Gm- and Gm+ infections.

MACROLIDE ANTIBIOTIC: ERYTHROMYCIN

Action: Bacteriostatic. Inhibits synthesis of protein in bacteria.

Indications: Clients who are allergic to penicillin. Gram-positive and some gram-negative organisms.

Warnings: Hepatic dysfunction, lactation.

Undesirable Effects: Low rate of undesirable effects. Anorexia, nausea, vomiting, diarrhea (usually dose related); tinnitus; rash.

Other Specific Information: ↑ effect of digoxin, carbamazepine, cyclosporine, theophylline, triazolam, warfarin. ↓ effect of clindamycin, penicillins.

Interventions: Periodic hepatic function studies for high-doses or prolonged IV therapy. Monitor bleeding times if taking warfarin. If administered IV, dilute in an appropriate amount of solution as outlined in the drug book or circular. (Refer to "**MEDICATE**".)

Education: Instruct client to take erythromycin 1 hour before or 2 hours after meals. Take with a full glass of water and not fruit juice. (Acids in fruit juices decrease the activity of the drug.) If GI upset occurs, client may take with food. Chewable tablets should be chewed and not swallowed. Report undesirable effects. (Refer to "**MEDICATE**".)

Evaluation: Negative cultures. Body temperature and WBC count will be within normal range.

Drugs: erythromycin (E-Mycin, Erytab, Eryc, PCE, Ilotycin, Ilosone, EES, EryPed, Erythrocin)

MACROLIDE GIRL

G I disturbances—undesirable effect

I V site—✔ for irritation

R educes activity of med if given
with acids (fruit juices) or food

L iver function tests

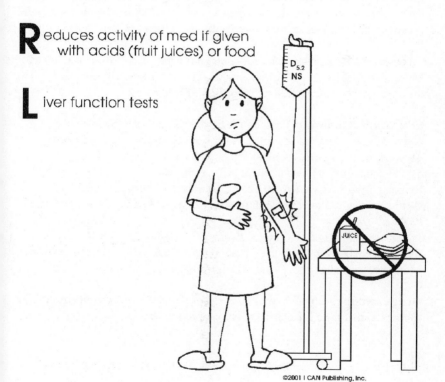

©2001 I CAN Publishing, Inc.

MACROLIDES

Action: Inhibits bacterial protein synthesis.

Indications: Gram positive bacteria with limited gram negative coverage. Uses include respiratory, gastrointestinal tract, skin and soft tissue infections when beta-lactam antibiotics are contraindicated.

Warnings: Hypersensitivity; hepatic / renal dysfunction.

Undesirable Effects: GI upset occurs in 20-30% of clients.

Other Specific Information: Theophyline, digoxin, carbamazepine, phenytoin, methylprednisolone, and warfarin can have ↑effects when taken with these macrolides. ↓ absorption with antacids. ↓ effect of clindamycin.

Interventions: Monitor liver function tests, vital signs, I & O. Maintain good hydration. Evaluate for blood dyscrasias (platelets) especially in long term use of azithromycin. (Refer to **"MEDICATE".**)

Education: Notify provider of rash or diarrhea. Drink fluids liberally. Azithromycin – take at least one hour prior to or 2 hours after a meal. Avoid giving with food. Avoid simultaneous administration of magnesium or aluminum – containing antacids. Clarithromycin – take without regard to meals. May take with milk. Do not refrigerate the suspension form. Dirithromycin – take with food or within 1 hour of eating. (Refer to **"MEDICATE".**)

Evaluation: Negative cultures. Body temperature, and WBC count will be within normal range.

Drugs: azithromycin (Zithromax); clarithromycin (Biaxin); dirithromycin (Dynabec); erythromycin (Refer to erythromycin)

ZEB

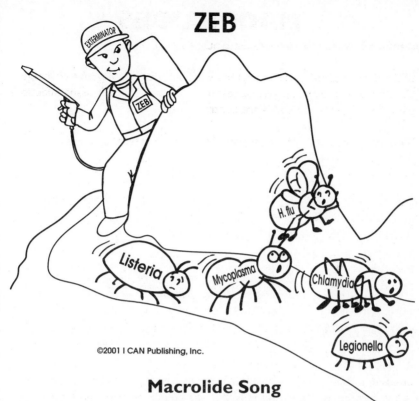

©2001 I CAN Publishing, Inc.

Macrolide Song

(sung to the tune of "She'll Be Coming Around the Mountain")

Chorus
One good bug exterminator—Macrolide
Zithromax, EES, Biaxin are the types.
But if used improperly
Major problems you might see
Always check your text and give it properly.

Verse 1
Contraindicated drugs with Macrolides
Dilantin toxicity, so don't you dare provide
And your blood will soon become too thin
If you take it with your Coumadin
So don't you mix these drugs and you'll
    survive.

Verse 2
Erythromycin and Biaxin Macrolides
Cause increased levels with carbamazepine
Hold Theophylline and Dig
Cause toxic affects will run real big
Solu Medrol is another risk besides.

Verse 3
If your poop runs and smells real bad
    on Macrolides
And girls taking these are scratching at
    their hides.
Or a black tongue that is furry
Call your provider in a hurry.
'Cuz a superinfection these are all the signs.

"ZEB" (Zithromax, Erythromycin, Biaxin) is one good bug exterminator.

PENICILLINS

Action: Bactericidal. Inhibits the enzyme in cell wall synthesis.

Indications: Most gram-positive and gram-negative cocci and bacilli. Pneumonia, respiratory disease, urinary tract infection, syphilis, gonorrhea, meningitis, skin infections, some bone and joint infections, catheter infections. Gram-negative organisms affecting gastrointestinal tract: Salmonella and Shigella.

Warnings: Hypersensitivity to penicillin or cephalosporins. Caution with renal failure, GI disease, bleeding disorders, or hepatic disorders.

Undesirable Effects: Nausea, vomiting, diarrhea, rash, stomatitis. Hypersensitivity ranging from rash, urticaria, pruritus to full anaphylaxis. Superinfection–signs and symptoms include black, furry tongue, thrush, and vaginal discharge. Hematologic effects and neurotoxicity may present in select drugs.

Other Specific Information: Decreased effect with tetracycline and erythromycin.

Interventions: Monitor WBCs, culture/sensitivity reports, I & O, renal function tests, liver enzymes, and temperature. (Sudden increase in temperature may indicate drug fever.) Benadryl may be given for mild reactions. Check for bleeding if high doses of penicillin are being given. Monitor for seizures in clients with renal disease. Dilute medicine for IV use in appropriate amount of solution. Refer to drug circular. (Refer to "**MEDICATE**".)

Education: Call provider immediately if rash, fever, chills, diarrhea, or bleeding occur. For best results take 1–2 hours before or 2–3 hours after meals. May take with food if problems occur with GI upset. Encourage client to increase fluids. Wear a med identification necklace or bracelet if any allergies.(Refer to "**MEDICATE**".)

Evaluation: Negative cultures. Body temperature and CBC, especially WBC count will be within normal range.

Drugs: *Broad spectrum:* amoxicillin (Amoxil, Polymax, Trimox, Wymox); amoxicillin/clavulanate (Augmentin); ampicillin (Omnipen, Polycillin); ampicillin/sulbactam (Unasyn); aztreonam (Azactam) bacampicillin (Spectrobid); *Extended spectrum:* carbenicillin (Geocillin); mezlocillin (Mezlin); piperacillin (Pipracil); piperacillin/tazobactum (Zosyn); ticarcillin (Ticar); ticarcillin/calvulanate (Timentin); *Naturals:* penicillin G benzathine (Bicillin, Permapen); penicillin G postassium (Pentids, Pfizerpen); penicillin G procaine (Crysticillin, A.S. Wycillin); penicillin V potassium (Pen-Vee K, V-Cillin K, Veetids); *Penicillinase resistant:* cloxacillin (Cloxapen, Tegopen); dicloxacillin (Dynapen, Pathocil); methicillin (Staphcillin); nafcillin (Nafcil, Unipen); oxacillin (Bactocill, Prostaphilin)

Anti-Infective Agents

PENICILLIN

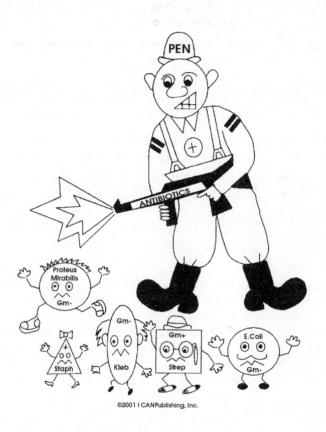

©2001 I CANPublishing, Inc.

PEN the antibiotic has his "destroyer laser" aimed at several types of bacteria. He is a broad spectrum antibiotic.

SULFONAMIDES

Action: Bacteriostatic. Interferes with bacterial growth by blocking folic acid synthesis in the cell.

Indications: Broad spectrum agents effective against gram-negative and gram-positive organisms. Urinary tract infection; respiratory infection; Pneumocystis carinii pneumonitis; acute otitis media; sinusitis; prostatitis; and gastrointestinal infections such as shigellosis, traveler's diarrhea prophylaxis.

Warnings: Hypersensitivity to trimethoprim or any sulfonamides. Megaloblastic anemia due to folate deficiency. Caution with elderly or renal/hepatic impairment.

Undesirable Effects: Anorexia, nausea/vomiting; rash; photosensitivity; acute hemolytic anemia and other blood dyscrasias; hepatic/renal toxicity; Steven-Johnson Syndrome (blistering and peeling of skin, arthralgia). Increased risk for bone marrow depression with the elderly client.

Other Specific Information: May ↑ effects of warfarin. Antacids ↓ absorption.

Interventions: Baseline hepatic, renal, and hematologic studies. Monitor I & O and vital signs at least twice a day. Adjust fluid intake to maintain output at least 1500 ml in 24 hours. (Refer to "**MEDICATE**".)

Education: Take orally with 8 oz. water; drink several extra glasses of fluids daily (unless contraindicated for renal or cardiac conditions). Administer 1 hour before or 2 hours after meals. If nausea and vomiting occur, administer with food. Avoid direct skin exposure to sun. Instruct clients with diabetes that sulfonamides may result in false-positive urine sugar and ketone test results. Report skin rash, cough, sore throat, sores in mouth, fever, bruising, or bleeding (early signs of blood dyscrasia). (Refer to "**MEDICATE**".)

Evaluation: Negative cultures. Body temperatue and WBC count will be within normal range.

Drugs: sulfadiazine (generic); sulfisoxazole (Gantrisin); trimethoprim - sulfamethoxazole (Bactrim, Septra)

SULFA

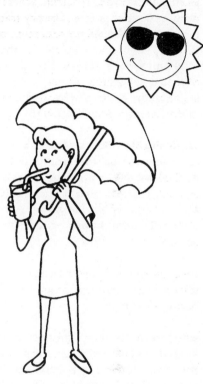

S unlight sensitivity—U E

U ndesirable effects—rash, renal toxicity

L ook for urine output, fever, sore throat and bleeding

©2001 I CAN Publishing, Inc.

F luids galore!

A norexia, anemia—U E

TETRACYCLINES

Action: Bacteriostatic. Inhibits protein synthesis by binding to ribosomes.

Indications: Gram-negative and gram-positive aerobes and anaerobes. Useful in treating skin infections, chlamydia, gonorrhea, syphilis, and atypical diseases such as Borrelia burghdorferi (Lyme disease), rickettsial diseases (Rocky Mountain Spotted Fever).

Warnings: Renal or hepatic dysfunction. Pregnant/breastfeeding women, and children less than 8 years of age due to permanent mottling and staining of teeth. The fetus or child may also experience a decrease in the linear skeletal growth rate. Caution with sun light exposure.

Undesirable Effects: Nausea, vomiting, diarrhea, dysphagia, abdominal cramping; rash; photosensitivity; nephrotoxicity (not as frequently with doxycycline); dental staining; superinfection (especially fungal).

Other Specific Information: Absorption impaired by milk, antacids, and iron. Tetracyclines may ↓ effectiveness of oral contraceptives. May alter effects of anticoagulants.

Interventions: Monitor liver enzymes, BUN, and serum creatinine. Monitor VS and urine output. Assess for rash and pattern of bowel activity. (Refer to "**MEDICATE**".)

Education: Instruct client to store medicine out of light and heat. Avoid excessive exposure to sunlight; photosensitivity may persist for some time after the drug has been discontinued. Take oral dose on empty stomach (1 hour before or 2 hours after food/beverage); drink full glass of water and avoid bedtime dose. Avoid antacids, dairy, and iron products. Advise that stools may be green or yellow. Topical application may cause skin to turn yellow. Recommend additional contraceptives and not to rely on oral contraceptives. (Refer to "**MEDICATE**".)

Evaluation: Client's body temperature, WBC count, and cultures will return to normal range.

Drugs: (*These drugs end in "cycline".*) demeclo**cycline** (Declomycin); doxy**cycline** (Vibramycin); mino**cycline** (Minocin); oxytetra**cycline** (Terramycin); tetra**cycline** (Achromycin)

TETRA"**CYCLINES**"

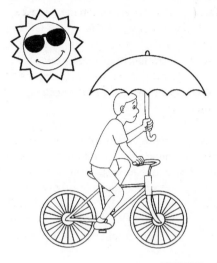
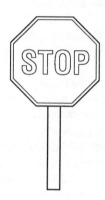

©2001 I CAN Publishing, Inc.

S unlight sensitivity

T ake with full glass of water

Ø antacid, iron, milk

P ut drug into empty stomach

"Trey" the cycler needs to STOP and go protect himself from the sun. "Stop" will help you remember how to safely take tetracyclines.

VANCOMYCIN HYDROCHLORIDE

Action: Bactericidal. Inhibits bacterial cell wall synthesis by binding to a cell wall precursor.

Indications: Antibiotic-associated pseudomembranous caused by Clostridium difficile and staphylococcal enterocolitis. Potentially life-threatening infections not responding to other less toxic antibiotics (parenteral).

Warnings: Renal failure, hearing loss, and concurrent use of other nephrotoxic/ototoxic drugs.

Undesirable effects: Nausea, vomiting, or taste alterations. Dose-related toxicity include tinnitus, high tone deafness, hearing loss, and nephrotoxicity. Rapid IV infusion can produce "red-neck or red man syndrome" resulting in histamine release and chills, fever, tachycardia, profound fall in BP, pruritus, or red face/neck/arms/back.

Other Specific Information: Aminoglycosides, amphotericin, aspirin, and furosemide may ↑ ototoxicity and/or nephrotoxicity.

Interventions: Check baseline hearing. Monitor blood pressure during administration. Monitor renal function tests and I & O. Monitor peak and trough levels. Draw trough level 30 minutes before the third dose is given. Monitor for "red-neck" syndrome. Stop infusion and report to provider of health care. Slowing the infusion or increasing the diluent volume may reduce "redneck" effect. Evaluate IV site for phlebitis. Avoid extravasation. (Refer to "**MEDICATE**.")

Education: Report ringing in ears or hearing loss, fever, and sore throat. Instruct that lab reports are a necessary part of the treatment. (Refer to "**MEDICATE**.")

Evaluation: Client's body temperature, WBC count, and cultures will return to normal range.

Drugs: vancomycin hydrochloride (Vancocin, Vancoled)

RUDOLPH THE
RED-NECK REINDEER

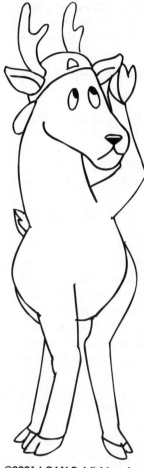

Rudolph the red-neck reindeer
Had an adverse side effect
From the drug Vancomycin,
Must keep all his labs in check.

Caution with renal failure,
Hearing loss and allergies,
Take a temp and blood cultures,
Especially that CBC!!!

©2001 I CAN Publishing, Inc.

CLINDAMYCIN

Action: Anti-infective. Binds to 50S subunit of bacterial ribosomes, suppresses protein synthesis.

Indications: Skin, skin structure, respiratory tract, intra-abdominal and gynecologic infections, septicemia, osteomyelitis, endocarditis prophylaxis, severe acne. Infections caused by staphylococci, streptococci, Rickettsia, Fusobacterium, Actinomyces, Peptococcus, Bacteroides, Pneumocystitis carinii.

Warnings: Hypersensitivity, history of pseudomembranous colitis, severe liver impairment, diarrhea.

Undesirable Effects: Arrhythmias, hypotension, pseudomembranous colitis, diarrhea, bitter taste (IV only).

Other Specific: Decreased absorption when taken with kaolin. May block clindamycin effect when taken with erythromycin. Increased neuromuscular blockade with neuromuscular blockers.

Interventions: Monitor GI status, diarrhea, abdominal cramping, fever, and bloody stools. These may be a sign of pseudomembranous colitis and should be reported immediately. Pseudomembranous colitis may begin up to several weeks following the cessation of therapy. Instruct client to finish the drug completely as directed, even if feeling better. Monitor liver studies, blood studies. Discontinue drug if bone marrow depression occurs. C&S prior to beginning medication. Monitor B/P, pulse in client receiving drug parenterally. Assess for skin irritation, dermatitis after administration. Assess respiratory status. Review potential allergies prior to beginning therapy. Administer with a glass of water; may be given with meals. IM—Do not administer >600 mg in a single IM injection. Intermittent Infusion: Rate: administer each 300 mg over a minimum of 10 min. If experiences an allergic reaction, withdraw drug immediately, maintain airway; administer epinephrine, aminophylline, O_2, IV corticosteroids.

Education: Advise to take po med with a full glass of water. May give with food to reduce GI symptoms. Discuss the importance of taking full course of medication. Report sore throat, fever, fatigue which may indicate a superinfection. Do not break, crush, or chew caps. Drug must be taken in equal intervals around the clock to maintain appropriate blood levels. Report any undesirable effects.

Evaluation: Client will have a normal temperature and a negative C&S.

Drug: clindamycin phosphate (Cleocin Phosphate, Dalacin C, Dalacin C Phosphate), clindamycin HCL (Cleocin HCl), clindamycin palmitate (Cleocin Pediatric, Dalacin C Palmitate)

CLINDAMYCIN

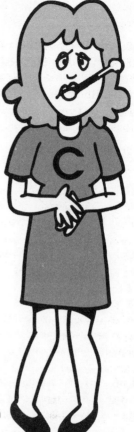

C olitis is a dangerous & life-threatening side effect

L iver function tests—monitor

I M injection limited to 600 mg, inject deep into large muscle to avoid problems

N euromuscular blockade increased with neuromuscular blockers

D iscontinue drug if bone marrow depression occurs

A rrhythmias—undesirable effects

©2005 I CAN Publishing, Inc.
"C LINDA" is sick and needs her **CLINDAMYCIN** to get well.

OXAZOLIDIN: ZYVOX

Action: Binds to bacterial 235 ribosomal RNA of the 50S subunit preventing formation of the bacterial translation process.

Indications: Vancomycin-resistant Enterococcus faecium infections, noscomial pneumonia, uncomplicated or complicated skin and skin structure infections, community-acquired pneumonia.

Warnings: Hypersensitivity. Thrombocytopenia.

Undesirable Effects: Headache, dizziness; nausea, diarrhea, increased ALT, AST, vomiting, taste change, tongue color change; vaginal moniliasis, fungal infection, oral moniliasis; myelosuppression.

Other Specific Information: May decrease the effects of MAOIs; increased effects of adrenergic agents, serotonergic agents.

Interventions: Assess CBC weekly, assess for myelosuppression (anemias, leukopenia, pancytopenia, thrombocytopenia). Assess for CNS symptoms such as headaches, dizziness; liver function tests: AST, ALT; allergic reactions; pseudomembranous colitis.

Education: Advise if dizziness occurs to ambulate, perform activities with assistance. Complete full course of med. Notify provider for any undesirable effects. Avoid large amounts of high-tyramine foods.

Evaluation: Decreased symptoms of infection, blood cultures negative.

Drug: linezolid (Zyvox)

ZYVOX

Z ero drug additives to IV line

^T**Y** ramine foods to be avoided

V RE and MRSA effective drug

O ral & IV use same dosages

^o**X** azolidin antibiotic

©2005 I CAN Publishing, Inc.

ANTITUBERCULAR: ISONIAZID

Action: Interferes with DNA synthesis.

Indications: Tuberculosis; prophylactic drug against tuberculosis.

Warnings: Alcoholism; renal or hepatic disease; diabetic retinopathy; pregnancy, lactation.

Undesirable Effects: Peripheral neuropathy; nausea, vomiting, hepatotoxicity.

Other Specific Information: ↑ risk of isoniazid-related hepatitis with alcohol, rifampin. ↑ drug levels of phenytoin, carbamazepine.

Interventions: Collect specimens for culture and sensitivity; sputum analysis; monitor hepatic function results, BUN, and serum creatinine. Assess for symptoms of peripheral neuropathy, such as tingling or numbness of the extremities. Administer pyridoxine (vitamin B_6) to any client who is high risk for developing peripheral neuropathy, such as malnourished, elderly, diabetic, or alcoholics.

Education: Take 1 hour before or 2 hours after meals; don't skip doses; take full length of therapy. Avoid sauerkraut, tuna, aged cheese, smoked fish (foods containing tyramine) that may cause reaction such as pounding heart, dizziness, clammy feeling, headache, red skin. Advise client not to drink alcohol and take meds without consulting provider. Recommend no antacids while taking drug. Instruct client regarding the importance of routine office visits for ongoing evaluation. Review plans for safety with machinery or driving. Notify provider of any undesirable effects.

Evaluation: Client will be free from infection and will have a negative sputum specimen for acid-fast bacilli.

Drugs: isoniazid (INH, Laniazid, Nydrazid)

INA TUBERCULOSIS

L iver enzymes—must be monitored

U se cautiously with renal dysfunction

N o alcohol

G ive pyridoxine (B$_6$)—prevent peripheral neuropathy

S hould take on empty stomach, screen vision

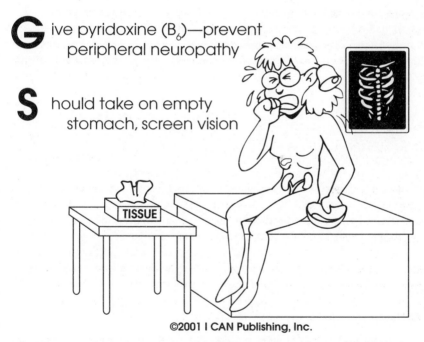

©2001 I CAN Publishing, Inc.

In some communities, Isoniazid (INH) has been nicknamed "INA". INA Tuberculosis has undesirable effects from INH. She is nauseated, has an enlarged liver, tingling in her feet (peripheral neuropathy), and her secretions have turned orange. "LUNGS" will help you recall some interventions.

ANTITUBERCULAR: RIFAMPIN

Action: Impairs RNA synthesis.

Indications: Treatment of pulmonary tuberculosis with at least one other antitubercular agent and for asymptomatic meningococcal carriers of Neisseria meningitidis.

Warnings: Hypersensitivity; hepatic dysfunction; active or treated alcoholism; children < than 5 years of age; pregnancy, lactation.

Undesirable Effects: Headache, drowsiness, dizziness; epigastric distress, heartburn, elevations of liver enzymes, hepatitis; rash and "flu-like syndrome" (chills, general discomfort, fever); blood dyscrasias; red-orange color to tears, saliva, sweat, urine, sputum. Soft contact lenses may be permanently stained.

Other Specific Information: When administered in combination with isoniazid, ↑ incidence of rifampin-related hepatitis. ↓ effectiveness of rifampin with ketoconazole. ↓ effectiveness of corticosteroids, metoprolol, propranolol, oral contraceptives, oral sulfonylureas, digitoxin, warfarin, etc. (*It is beyond the scope of this book to review all of the interactions. Refer to Drug Handbook.*)

Interventions: Monitor hepatic and renal function tests, CBC, cultures, sputum analysis, and urinalysis. Monitor CBC results for dyscrasias and observe for infection, hemorrhaging, or unusual fatigue. Arrange for a follow up with an ophthalmologist. If client is unable to swallow, recommend a suspension.

Education: Instruct not to skip dose; do not stop this drug without consulting with provider of care. Advise to take on empty stomach 1 hr. before or 2 hrs. after meals. Advise no alcohol or other meds without consulting provider. Take rifampin at least one hour before antacid. Advise client that urine and secretions may turn red-orange; do not wear soft contact lenses while taking this drug. Notify provider of any undesirable effects. If taking oral contraceptives, recommend alternative birth control. Recommend that client avoid activities that require alertness until response has been determined.

Evaluation: Client will be free of infection with no undesirable effects from the medicine.

Drug: rifampin (Rifadin, Rimactane)

REDMAN RIFAMPIN

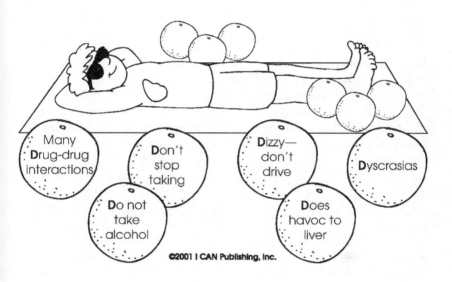

Many **D**rug-drug interactions

Don't stop taking

Do not take alcohol

Dizzy— don't drive

Does havoc to liver

Dyscrasias

©2001 I CAN Publishing, Inc.

Meet Mr. Redman Rifampin. He is taking some r & r (rest and relaxation) and is at the beach eating many oranges. He has had so many oranges his pee and tears are orange. Rifampin is hard on the liver, so it has gotten larger. The oranges will help you recall the 6 D's of rifampin.

ANTIFUNGAL: AMPHOTERICIN B

Action: Alters fungal cell permeability

Indications: Systemic fungal infections such as histoplasmosis or coccidioidomycosis.

Warnings: Hypersensitivity. Renal impairment, in combination with antineoplastic therapy. Pregnancy / Lactation.

Undesirable Effects: Very toxic. Infusion-related reaction (fever, chills, nausea, vomiting, headache, hypotension); drying effect with skin, pruritus; nephrotoxicity; thrombophlebtis; anemia; hypokalemia; ventricular fibrillation.

Other Specific Information: Steroids may ↑risk of severe hypokalemia. May ↑digoxin toxicity. Bone marrow depressants may ↑anemia. Nephrotoxic drugs may ↑nephrotoxicity.

Intervention: Monitor I & O, renal function tests for nephrotoxicity, and hepatic function test results. Evaluate potassium and magnesium levels, and hematologic results. Monitor vital signs and assess for undesirable effects q 15 min x 2, then q 30 min for 4 hrs. of initial infusion. Administer Tylenol and Benedryl 1 hour before infusion. Add hydrocortisone to infusion. Observe for signs of hypokalemia (muscle cramps, irregular pulse, and weakness). Large doses of potassium may be needed. Evaluate IV site for phlebitis. If client experiences GI symptoms, a pleasant and relaxed atmosphere for mealtimes along with small, frequent feedings of high-protein, high-calorie foods should be encouraged.

Education: Review oral hygiene such as using soft toothbrushes and floss. Avoid toothpicks. Advise client to notify staff at the first sign of pain at IV site. Report undesirable effects immediately to staff.

Evaluation: The client's infection will be eradicated without undesirable effects from the medication.

AMPHOTERRIBLE

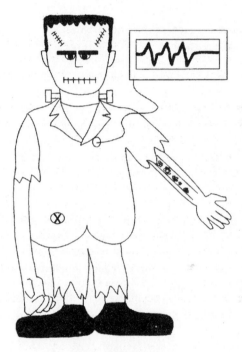

©2001 I CAN Publishing, Inc.

Ampho**terrible** is a monster. He treats monster infections such as histoplasmosis and other life threatening fungal infections. He has a terrible habit of creating irregularities in the heart (arrhythmias). The X marks the spot of the kidney since 80% of clients receiving this drug may develop some nephrotoxicity.

ANTIFUNGALS

Action: Increases permeability of the fungal cell membrane causing cell death.

Indications: Fungal infections: candidiasis, coccidioidomycosis, histo-plasmosis, ringworm infections of the skin, tinea corporis, tinea cruris, onchomycosis of nails.

Warnings: Hypersensitivity to any antifungal, liver failure, pregnancy, lactation.

Undesired Effects: Headache, dizziness; nausea, vomiting, pruritus, irritation with topical application.

Other Specific Information: ↓ blood levels with rifampin. ↑ risk of toxicity of cyclosporine with antifungals. ↑ length of suppression of the adrenal cortex when corticosteroids or methylprednisolone are taken with antifungals. Risk of arrhythmias and even death when given with antihistamines.

Interventions: Evaluate liver function tests, CBC and differential, and culture the area prior to starting therapy; LFT may be done monthly. If a severe allergic reaction occurs, have epinephrine available.

Education: Instruct client to take medication with food; provide small frequent meals if GI upset is present. Review importance of taking the full course of medication. If no improvement within 2 wks, notify provider. Discuss hygiene measures to control reinfection. Review safety precautions if dizziness occurs.

Evaluation: Client's fungal infection will be resolved as indicated by a decrease in pruritus, redness, and rawness.

Drugs: *(Many of these drugs end in "zole".)* amphotericin B; fluconazole (Diflucan); flucystosine (Ancobon); itraconazole (Sporanox); ketoconazole (Nizoral); miconazole (Monistat IV); nystatin (Nilstat, Nystex); *Vaginal sup-positories, topical:* miconazole (Micatin, Monistat 3, Monistat 7, Monistat-Derm, Monistat Dual Pak); nystatin (Mycostatin); *Topical:* butenafine (Mentax); butoconazole (Femstat 3); ciclopirox (Penlac); clotrimazole (Lotrimin, Mycelex); econazole (Spectazole); gentian violet; nafitine (Naftin); oxiconazole (Oxistat); terbinafine (Lamisil); tolnaftate (Aftate, Genaspor, Tinactin, Ting)

ZOLE

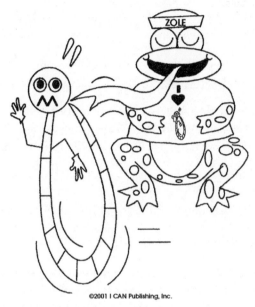

©2001 I CAN Publishing, Inc.

Z OLE—many drug interactions can occur

O bserve hygiene measures to control infection

L iver Function Tests—monitor

E ducate to take with food

Meet "ZOLE" the toad who destroys fungal infections, such as ringworm. "ZOLE" will help you remember some key points with these drugs. It will also help you remember the medication used for these infections, since they have the letters **zole** in them.

ANTIPROTOZOAL, AMEBICIDE: FLAGYL

Action: Inhibits DNA synthesis in specific anaerobes resulting in cell death. Antiprotozoal-trichomonacidal; amebicidal.

Indications: Trichomoniasis; Gardnerella vaginalis; amebic liver abscess; intestinal amebiasis.

Warnings: Hypersensitivity, blood dyscrasias, CNS diseases, candidiasis, hepatic disease, pregnancy, lactation.

Undesirable Effects: Headache, dizziness, ataxia; anorexia, nausea, vomiting, diarrhea, unpleasant metallic taste; dryness and burning skin; superinfection (candidiasis); disulfiram-like interaction with alcohol.

Other Specific Information: ↓ effectiveness with barbiturates. ↑ bleeding tendencies with oral anticoagulants. If taken with alcohol, client will experience flushing, nausea, increased vomiting, and tachycardia.

Interventions: Monitor CBC and liver function tests.

Education: Instruct to take full course of medication; take with food. Encourage mouth care, sugarless candies, etc. to assist with dry mouth. No alcohol or preparation containing alcohol during therapy and for at least 48 hours afterward. Inform that brown urine may occur. No intercourse unless partner wears a condom. Review undesirable effects and the importance of reporting them to provider. For the topical application, recommend cleaning area and waiting 15 to 20 minutes before applying drug. Avoid eye contact. Cosmetics may be used after applying drug.

Evaluation: Client will maintain an infection free state with no undesirable effects from the drug.

Drugs: metronidazole (Flagyl, Flagyl ER, Flagyl IV, MetroGel)

FLAGYL

F lushing

A LCOHOL will cause these effects

I ncreased vomiting

N ausea

T achycardia

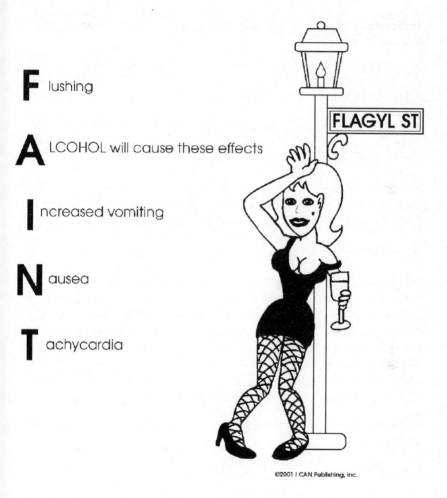

FLAGYL ST

©2001 I CAN Publishing, Inc.

As you can see, this lady has been doing her tricks on Flagyl Street. She evidently had alcohol while on this street. If Flagyl is mixed with alcohol, there will be a disulfiram-like reaction, and that is why this lady feels "FAINT".

ANTIVIRALS

Action: Interfere with DNA synthesis and replication of virus. Virustatic.

Indications: Herpes simplex I, genital herpes II.

Warnings: Hypersensitivity to any component of product. Caution with pregnancy/lactation, renal/hepatic impairment.

Undesirable Effects: Anorexia, nausea, vomiting; light-headedness, headaches, tremors; rash, pruritus. Increased bleeding time; phlebitis at IV site. Acyclovir–(Serious) nephrotoxicity, neuropathy, bone marrow depression.

Other Specific Information: Probenecid may ↑ acyclovir and valacyclovir levels. Increase nephroneurotoxicity when aminoglycosides, probenecid, and interferon are adminstered with acyclovir. None significant for famciclovir.

Interventions: Monitor renal/liver function tests, CBC, I & O, and vital signs (especially blood pressure). Acyclovir may cause orthostatic hyptension. Evaluate for superinfection due to high dose and prolonged use of an antiviral drug. If giving acyclovir IV, never give as a bolus. Refer to drug circular for specific guidelines. Provide analgesics and comfort measures to elderly with shingles. Keep fingernails short and clean.

Education: Review importance of fluid intake. Notify provider if condition worsens. Review ways to control spread. Teach to use finger cot or rubber glove when applying ointment to prevent spread of lesions. These meds do not cure herpes; they only shorten the episode. Pap smears should be done at least annually due to increased risk of cervical cancer in women with genital herpes. Avoid sexual intercourse during treatment for genital herpes.

Evaluation: Client will experience a decrease in the symptoms of the virus with no undesirable effects from the medications.

Drugs: (*end in "vir"*) acyclo**vir** (Zovirax); famciclo**vir** (Famvir); valacyclo**vir** (Valtrex)

THE VIR HOUSE OF SHINGLES

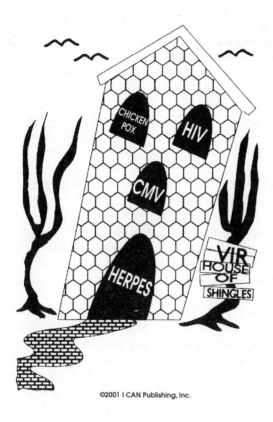

©2001 I CAN Publishing, Inc.

The haunted house of shingles (herpes zoster), chicken pox (varicella zoster), herpes simplex, and the cytomegaly virus is most often repaired with drugs that include **VIR** in them. Acyclo**vir** (Zo**vir**ax), famciclo**vir** (Fam-**vir**), and valacyclo**vir** (Valtrex) are a few of these drugs.

The house is haunted and shaky because the recipient of these drugs may experience a headache and shakes from chills. It's enough to make you throw up!

URINARY AGENT: PYRIDIUM

Action: Exact mechanism is not understood. Produces a topical analgesic effect on the urinary tract mucosa from the azo dye that is excreted.

Indications: Symptomatic relief of pain, burning, frequency related to irritation from a UTI.

Warnings: Hypersensitivity to phenazopyridine; renal insufficiency; pregnancy, lactation.

Undesirable Effects: Refer to "**GUSH**". **G**I disturbances, **U**rine may have a yellow-orange discoloration, **S**clera or skin may have a yellowish tinge, **H**emolytic anemia, headache.

Other Specific Information: May interfere with urinalysis color reactions, urinary ketones, glucose, proteins, and steroids.

Interventions: With long-term therapy, assess liver function tests. Do not administer longer than 2 days if given with antibacterial agent for the treatment of UTI. Discontinue drug if sclera or skin become yellowish; this indicates accumulation of drug.

Education: Instruct client to take after meals to decrease gastric irritation. Advise client that urine may be reddish-orange and may stain fabric. Report signs of yellowing of skin or sclera, headache, clay-colored stools, unusual bleeding or bruising, fever, sore throat.

Evaluation: Client will be free of pain from urinary tract in 3 days.

Drug: phenazopyridine (Pyridium)

MR. P.O.

GI disturbances

Urine turns yellow orange

Sclera and skin orange

Hemolytic anemia

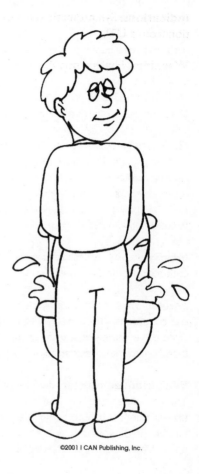

©2001 I CAN Publishing, Inc.

Mr. P.O. was not happy with his pain, but after taking Pyridium the pain from his UTI must be gone. Judging by the look on his face, Pyridium is obviously working. He can now pee out a "GUSH" without discomfort. Remember: **P**yridium turns urine **O**range!

PROTEASE INHIBITORS

Action: Inhibits the binding of the enzyme protease, which is needed for the HIV protein to mature. These agents act only during viral replication. Antiretroviral.

Indications: HIV infection. May be combined with nucleoside or reverse transcriptase inhibitors.

Warnings: Use cautiously with clients who have liver impairment. Interactions include toxicity of drugs activated by CYP3A4 (a liver enzyme).

Undesirable Effects: Kidney stones; GI symptoms: abdominal pain, diarrhea, nausea and vomiting, and altered sense of taste. *Neurologic:* headache, insomnia, weakness.

Other Specific Information: Never give at the same time as didanosine (Videx).

Interventions: Assess for signs of infection or anemia. Monitor AST, ALT. Culture and sensivity before drug therapy and after treatment. Assess bowel pattern during treatment. Assess urine color, consistency, and ease in urinating. Monitor skin eruptions, rash, urticaria. Monitor CD4 cell count throughout treatment. Administer with food. Do not mix with juice or acidic fluids. Administer antiemetic, antidiarrheal as needed. Implement safety measures in case of weakness. Encourage sedatives and nonopoid analgesics as needed.

Education: Avoid other medications unless directed by provider of care. The drug does not cure, but does manage symptoms and does not prevent transmission of HIV to others. Recommend to use a nonhormonal form of birth control while taking the drug. If miss dose take as soon as remembered up to 1 hour before next dose; do not double dose. Take with food.

Evaluation: Client will have a therapeutic effect from the medication with no complications from undesirable effects.

Drugs: indinavir (Crixivan), nelfinavir (Viracept), ritonavir (Norvir), saquinavir (Invirase)

PECANS

P rotease enzyme is inhibited which is needed for HIV protein to mature. These agents act only during viral replication.

E ncourage sedatives and nonopioid analgesics as needed

C autiously use with liver impairment

A bdominal pain, nausea and vomiting
ltered sense of taste—undesirable effects
dminister antiemetic and antidiarrheal as needed

N eurological side effects: headache, insomnia, weakness

S tones, kidney—monitor

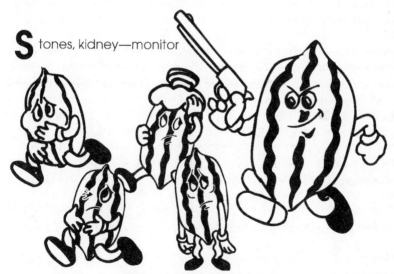

©2005 I CAN Publishing, Inc.

The chief PECAN is shooting to inhibit the binding of the enzyme protease. Note: This prevents maturity of the HIV protein.

NUCLEOSIDE INHIBITORS

Actions: Inhibits reverse transcriptase, that is needed to convert RNA into DNA in HIV infecion. HIV is a retrovirus, meaning that the genetic code is introduced opposite of a human gene (DNA to RNA).

Indications: HIV infections, both early onset and advanced stages. Lower transmission of HIV from mother to fetus.

Other Specific Information: Interactions can occur with other bone marrow depressants and certain antibiotics. Toxicity that occurs from the drugs may be difficult to distinguish from the symptoms of HIV infection.

Warnings: Hypersensitivity. Severe renal disease, impaired hepatic disease,

Undesirable Effects: Granulocytopenia and anemia; neurotoxicity: headache, insomnia, muscle pain, and nausea. Overdose: anemia, fatigue, leukopenia, severe nausea, thrombocytopenia, vomiting, seizures.

Interventions: Monitor CBC count. Perform a baseline neurologic assessment and check periodically thereafter. Monitor the effectiveness of the drug and the amount taken.

Education: Teach that drug is not a cure for AIDS but will control symptoms. Notify provider of care of sore throat, swollen lymph nodes, malaise, fever; other infections. Inform client that infection is still present and can be transmitted to others. Follow up visits must be continued since serious toxicity may occur; blood counts must be done q 2 weeks. Serious interactions may occur, so no OTC meds unless provider is aware.

Evaluation: Client will receive a therapeutic response from medication. Client will not experience any blood dyscrasias (anemia, granulocytopenia). Lab reports will remain with in the normal range.

Drugs: didanosine (Videx), lamivudine (Epivir), stavudine (Zerit), zalcitabine (HIVID), zidovudine (Retrovir)

REVERSE

R everse transcriptase is inhibited, which is needed to convert RNA into DNA in HIV infections. HIV is a retrovirus, meaning that the genetic code is introduced opposite of a human gene.

E valuate CBC

V ID or **VIR** are typically in the drug name (i.e., Retro**vir**, **Vid**ex, Epi**vir**, Hi**vid**)

E valuate neurological status

R eacts with bone marrow depressants and certain antibiotics

S ide effects—granulocytopenia and anemia, headache, insomnia, nausea

E valuate for overdose; some clients use as a suicide attempt (anemia, fatigue, leukopenia, thrombocytopenia, vomiting, seizures)

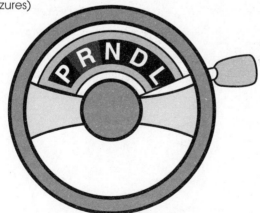

©2005 I CAN Publishing, Inc.

The steering wheel has been **reversed**. "REVERSE" will assist in recalling the most important facts about this category of drugs.

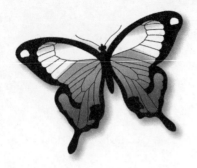

think ones' feelings waste themselves in words, they ought
all to be distilled into actions and into actions which bring
results.

Florence Nightingale

Antineoplastic Agents

UNDESIRABLE EFFECTS FROM ANTICANCER DRUGS

Bone marrow depression

Alopecia

Retching—nausea/vomiting

Fear and anxiety

Stomatitis

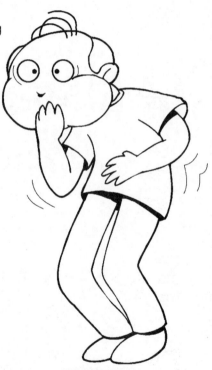

©2001 I CAN Publishing, Inc.

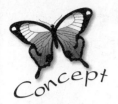

Concept

ANTINEOPLASTIC AGENTS

C B C, platelets—monitor

A ntiemetics before drug

N ephrotoxicity—undesirable effect

C ounseling regarding reproduction issues

E ncourage handwashing, avoid crowds

R ecommend a wig for alopecia

©2001 I CAN Publishing, Inc.

ALKYLATING AGENTS

Action: Causes cell death or mutation of malignant growths through inhibition of protein synthesis by interfering with DNA replication by alkylation of DNA. Action most evident in rapidly dividing cells.

Indications: Palliative treatment of chronic lymphocytic leukemia; malignant lymphomas; Hodgkin's disease; breast, lung and ovarian cancers.

Warnings: Hypersensitivity; bone marrow depression; active infections; recent immunization with live virus; renal or liver disease; concurrent radiation therapy; pregnancy, lactation.

Undesirable Effects: Tremors, muscular twitching, confusion; nausea, vomiting, hepatotoxicity; bone marrow depression; sterility; alopecia, urticaria; hemorrhagic cystitis; cancer, acute leukemia.

Other Specific Information: Individual drugs have specific interactions with meds. It is beyond the scope of this book to review.

Interventions: Monitor CBC with differential and platelets weekly. Monitor uric acid, liver and renal function tests before and throughout therapy. Hydrate client well before and after treatment. Premedicate with antietemics, ondansetron or granisetron are preferred. Have prn antiemetics available. Monitor IV site for irritation and phlebitis. Have epinephrine, corticosteroids, antihistamines and emergency equipment on hand for potential allergic reaction. Store drug in airtight container at room temperature.

Education: Consult with provider prior to receiving any vaccination. Instruct to report bleeding, signs of anemia, or infection to provider. Recommend a diet low in purines to alkalize urine. Review the importance of good oral hygiene with soft toothbrush. Do not use toothbrush when platelet count is <50,000 cells/mm^3. Reduce nausea and vomiting by eating small meals and refer for dietary consultation. (Refer to "**CANCER**".)

Evaluation: Client will be free of cancer; blood counts will improve.

Drugs: busulfan (Busulfex, Myleran); carboplatin (Paraplatin); carmustine (BiCNU, Gliadel); chlorambucil (Leukeran); cisplatin (Platinol-AQ); cyclophosphamide (Cytoxan, Neosar); ifosfamide (Ifex); lomustine (CeeNU); mechlorethamine (Mustargen); melphalan (Alkeran); streptozocin (Zanosar); thiotepa (Thioplex)

NITROGEN MUSTARD

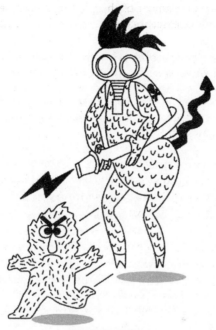

©2001 I CAN Publishing, Inc.

B one marrow depression (leukopenia, thrombocytopenia)

A norexia/alopecia

D istressful nausea and vomiting

Nitrogen Mustard, the alkylating agent, is destroying malignant neoplasm. Somewhat of a beast itself, it causes "**BAD**" undesirable effects.

ANTIMETABOLITES

Action: Interferes with the building blocks of DNA synthesis, greatest activity is in the S phase of the cell cycle.

Indications: Myelocytic leukemia; acute lymphocytic leukemia; cancer of breast, cervix, colon, liver, ovary, pancreas, stomach, and rectum; combination treatment for non-Hodgkin's lymphoma in children.

Warnings: Allergy; myelosuppression; active infections; recent immunization with live virus; renal or hepatic disease; pregnancy, lactation.

Undesirable Effects: Anorexia, nausea, vomiting, diarrhea, oral and anal inflammation; bone marrow depression, thrombocytopenia, hemorrhage; alopecia, rash, fever; renal dysfunction.

Other Specific Information: ↓ effect of digoxin with cytarbine. ↑ toxicity of fluorouracil with leucovorin. May be fatal if methotrexate is taken with specific NSAIDs. Interactions may occur with live virus vaccines, bone marrow depressants, calcium, and cimetidine.

Interventions: Evaluate complete blood count, uric acid, kidney and liver chemistries before administration. Evaluate neurological status prior to and during therapy. Premedicate with antiemetics. Comfort measures if headache, inflammation, or other associated pain occurs with cytarabine syndrome. Safety measures if dizziness occurs. (Refer to "**METABOLITE**" on next page.)

Education: Client should report fever, sore throat, extreme fatigue, rash, ulcers, tarry stools, bleeding, or other unusual symptoms to provider. Do not use a toothbrush if platelet count is <50,000/mm^3. Reduce nausea and vomiting by eating small meals and refer for dietary consultation. (Refer to "**CANCER**" and "**METABOLITE**".)

Evaluation: Client's tumor will decrease in size and blood tests will remain in normal range.

Drugs: capecitabine (Xeloda); cytarabine (Ara-C, Cytosar-U, DepoCyt, Tarabine PFS); floxuridine (FUDR); fludarabine (Fludara); fluorouracil (Adrucil, Efudex, Fluoroplex, 5-FU); mercaptopurine (Purinethol); methotrexate (MTX); thioguanine (6-Thioguanine)

ANTIMETABOLITE

M onitor CBC and platelets weekly

E valuate renal function tests

T emperature assessment q 4–6 hrs.

A sepsis—strict

B leeding, anemia, infection, and nausea—report

O ral hygiene—brush with soft toothbrush

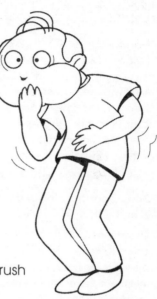

©2001 I CAN Publishing, Inc.

L ots of fluids (2–3 L/day)

I ntake and Output, nutritional intake—monitor

T he Protocols for handling and administering—follow

E mphasize protective isolation

ANTINEOPLASTIC AGENTS: ANTIBIOTICS

Action: Inhibits RNA synthesis and delays or inhibits mitosis. Interferes with DNA replication and messenger RNA production.

Indications: Most useful in treating slow growing tumors. Hodgkin's disease, testicular carcinoma, breast and bladder cancer.

Warnings: **HIGH ALERT DRUG** Hypersensitivites. Use cautiously with client who have cardiopulmonary disease, dose reduction may be necessary. Caution in client with depressed bone marrow function, active infections, recent immunization with live virus, impaired renal or hepatic function, history of cardiopulmonary disease or diminished cardiac function. Use with caution for those with antineoplastic or radiation therapy within 3–6 weeks. Dactinomycin is contraindicated for clients with viral infections. This drug should be used with caution for obese clients or those with gout.

Undesirable Effects: Most antitumor antibiotics are toxic to the heart and lungs.

Other Specific Information: Increased toxicity with other antineoplastics or radiation. Alopecia, stomatitis, nausea, and vomiting are the most commonly occurring nonorgan-specific undesirable effects. Daunorubicin and doxorubicin may cause dose-limiting myelosuppression.

Interventions: All are vesicants except bleomycin. Severe tissue damage if extravasation. Administer with precautions to avoid tissue damage. Avoid with live vaccines. Monitor the CBC. Evaluate the client's cardiac and pulmonary status prior to and during treatment.. Administer antiemetics before initiating therapy and provide with antiemetics for home use.

Education: When reconstituted, daunorubicin and doxorubicin have a bright, reddish-orange color, which causes the client's urine to turn a similar color. Dactinomycin is a radiation sensitizer and may cause a phenomenon called radiation recall. This condition means that tissue that was damaged by radiation may become reddened and inflamed in response to antineoplastic therapy. Provide comprehensive client education on management of the symptoms and when to seek medical support.

Evaluation: The client will experience a therapeutic effect from the drug. There will be a decreased tumor size and a decrease in the spread of the malignancy.

Drugs: bleomycin (Blenoxane), dactinomycin (Cosmegen), daunorubicin (DaunoXome), doxorubicin (Adriamycin PFS, Adriamycin RDF, Rubex), epirubicin (Ellence), idarubicin (Idamycin, Idamycin PFS), methotrexate (Folex, Folex PFS, methotrexate, Rheumatrex), mitomycin (Mitomycin, Mutamycin), mitoxantrone (Novantrone), plicamycin (Mithramycin, Mithracin)

CINEMANS

C olor of urine changes

I ncreased opportunistic infection

N ausea and vomiting

E xtravasation

M yelosuppression, mucositis

A lopecia

N ausea and vomiting

S terility

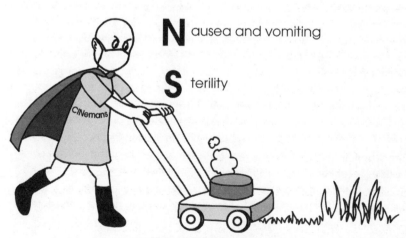

©2005 I CAN Publishing, Inc.

Mr. "CINemans" is mowing away at the slow growing weeds (cancer cells). Many of these agents end in "CIN"!

MITOTIC INHIBITORS

Action: Inhibits cell mitosis

Indications: Breast cancer, lymphomas, leukemia, Wilm's tumor, sarcomas

Warnings: Hypersensitivity; Paclitaxel (Taxol) is contraindicated for clients with a neutropenia count of less than 1500 cells/mm3. It is also used with caution in clients with cardiac dysrhythmias. Etoposide (VP-16) is contraindicated for clients with severe bone marrow depression, current or recent infection, and severe renal and hepatic dysfunction. Used with caution for clients with gout. Women during pregnancy; during lactation; and for children. Vincristine should be used cautiously in clients with infection, leukopenia, bone marrow suppression, chickenpox, current neurologic or neuromuscular hepatic dysfunction.

Undesirable Effects: Allergic interactions since all are plant derivatives. All of the vinca alkaloids are vesicants, which means that these drugs are capable of causing permanent tissue damage and necrosis when allowed to extravasate into tissues. VIncristine is fatal if given intrathecally.

Other Specific Information: When vinblastine is given concurrently with mitomycin, bronchospasms may occur. When paclitaxel and ketoconazole are given together, serious toxicities may occur.

Interventions: When giving vesicant drugs via a peripheral IV route, extreme caution must be taken to establish a reliable IV access that has not been subjected to a recent venipuncture. Vinca alkaloids (vesicant drugs) can cause leakage of drug into soft tissues around the venipuncture site (extravasation). Remember "V" for vesicant and use precautions with Velban, Vincristine, Vinblastine, Vindesine. Establish a protocol for administration of antidotes and application of heat or cold before administering a vesicant drug. Administer antidotes to minimize the damage caused by extravasation. Verify that informed consent has been given before initiating treatment. Check the client's lab and diagnostic studies before beginning therapy with special attention being given to the CBC, platelet count, and liver function studies. Monitor for bone marrow depression and peripheral neuropathy.

Education: Instruct client about signs and symptoms of peripheral neuropathy, including paresthesias in the hands or feet, difficulty with fine-motor skills, and numbness. Other signs and symptoms include constipation, paralytic ileus, urinary retention, and jaw pain. Instruct client to report any of these complaints immediately to the health care provider. (Failure to report peripheral neuropathy immediately may result in irreversible neurological damage.)

Evaluation: Client's cancer will decrease and blood tests will remain in normal range.

Drugs: Etoposide (VP-16), Paclitaxel (Taxol), Vinblastine (Velban), Vincristine (Oncovin), vinorelbine (Navelbine)

MITOTIC INHIBITOR: ANTINEOPLASTIC AGENTS

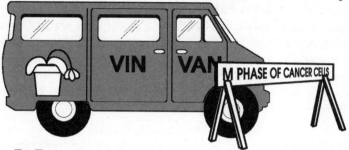

M ay cause hepatotoxicty

I nhibits cell mitosis

T ake precautions—vesicants (remember V's for vesicant: Vincristine, Vinblastine, Velban)

O ncovin (Vincristine)

T reat for breast cancer, lymphomas, leukemia, Wilm's Tumor

Rev **I** ew client's mobility and ADLs

C NS and neuro side effects such as peripheral neuropathy

©2005 I CAN Publishing, Inc.

The "VIN VAN" will help you remember that several of these agents start with "VIN". These agents block cell mitosis.

BIOLOGICAL RESPONSE MODIFIER
(Interferon)

Action: Possess antiviral and antineoplastic effects, directly inhibit effects on DNA and protein synthesis, and increase cancer cell antigens on the cell surface. This enables the immune system to recognize the cancer cells more easily. These actions halt virus replication and prevent penetration into healthy cells. They enhance the activity of the other cells in the immune system and stop the division of the cancer cells.

Indications: Treatment of viral infections: rhinovirus, papillovirus, tetrovirus, hepatitis, chondyloma—a wart-like growth in the perineal area; transmitted sexually. Treatment of various cancers: Kaposi's sarcoma, mulitple myeloma, renal cell carcinoma, melanoma, bladder cancer, T-cell lymphoma. Treatments of some autoimmune diseases: multiple sclerosis.

Warnings: Allergies to egg protein or neomycin. If allergic, do not adminiter these agents. Hypersensitivity. Renal, cardiac, or hepatic disease.

Undesirable Effects: Flu-like symptoms: fever, chills, headache, malaise, myalgia, and fatigue. *GI:* nausea, vomiting, diarrhea, anorexia. *CNS:* dizzy, confusion, paranoia. *CV:* tachycardia, cyanosis, tachypnea. *Hematologic* neutropenia, thrombocytopenia. Renal: increased BUN and creatinine levels, proteinuria, and altered LFTs.

Other Specific Information: Interactions can occur with aminophylline therapy, and there are additive effects with other antiviral agents

Interventions: Determine if there are any egg allergies. If severe, do not start therapy. If reaction is mild, then give antihistamines and begin therapy. Monitor CBC, renal studies. Monitor vital signs. Assess for signs of bleeding and infections. Implement safety precautions if CNS effects occur. Use nonopoid analgesics prn for flulike symptoms.

Education: Discuss the importance for reporting any bleeding or signs of infection. Review safety precautions with client for both bleeding and infection. Provide client and/or family written directions regarding how to take medication safely.

Evaluation: Client will experience decreased serious infections, improvement in existing infections and inflammatory conditions.

Drugs: interferon-alfa (Roferon-A, Alferon N), interferon-beta (Betaseron), interfeon-gamma (Actimmune)

Antineoplastic Agents

INTERFERON

F lu-like effect

E valuate for bleeding, ↑HR, ↑RR

V ertigo

E gg allergies

R eview CBC, BUN, creatinine

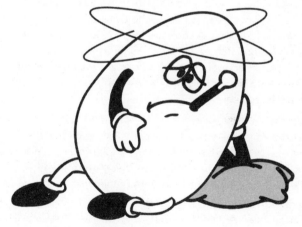

©2005 I CAN Publishing, Inc.

The sick Mr. Egg is reminding us not to administer these agents if client has any egg allergies. "FEVER" will help you remember some undesirable effects from these agents.

ANTI-ESTROGEN
TAMOXIFEN

Action: Antineoplastic. Antiestrogen homone. Inhibits cell division by binding to cytoplasmic estrogen receptors; resembles normal cell complex but inhibits DNA synthesis and estrogen response of target tissue.

Indications: Advanced breast carcinoma not responsive to other therapy in estrogen-receptor-positive patients (usually post menopausal), prevention of breast cancer, following breast surgery/radiation in ductal carcinoma in situ.

Warnings: Hypersensitivity; Leukopenia, thrombocytopenia, cataracts.

Undesirable Effects: Thrombocytopenia, leukopenia, vaginal bleeding, DVT, PE, nausea, vomiting, anorexia, rash, alopecia, hot flashes, headache, light-headedness, depression. Visual acuity may be decreased and the loss is irreversible.

Other Specific Information: Increased chance of bleeding when taken with anticoagulants. Bromocriptine may increase tamoxifen levels.

Interventions: Assess CBC, differential, platelet count every week; hold drug if WBC<3500 or platelet count is <100,000; notify provider of care. Assess for bleeding q 8 hours: hematuria, guaiac, bruising, petechiae, mucosa or orifices. Assess for psychological effects to the alopecia. Assess for symptoms indicating severe allergic reactions: rash, pruritus, urticaria, purpuric skin lesions, itching, flushing. Administer antacid prior to the oral agent; administer after evening meal, before going to bed. Administer an antiemetic 30–60 min. before giving drug to prevent vomiting. Do not crush, break, or chew tablets.

Education: Review importance of a liquid diet, if necessary, including cola, jello; dry toast or crackers if client is having difficulties with nausea and vomiting. Advise client to increase fluid intake to 2–3 L/day to prevent dehydration. Discuss taking in a nutritious diet with iron and vitamin supplements as ordered. Store in a light-resistant container at room temperature. Review the undesirable effects with the client and family members and advise to report to provider of care. Apply sunscreen and protective clothes when out in the sun. Report any vaginal bleeding immediately. Routine eye exams. Premenopausal women must use mechanical birth control because ovulation may be induced. Advise that new hair growth may be different in color and texture.

Evaluation: The client will have a decrease in the tumor size or spread of malignancy.

Drugs: tamoxifen (Tamoxifen, Nolvadex, Tamofen, Tamoplex, Tamone)

"TAMI OX SUN"

T hrombocytopenia, leukopenia, visual acuity
   decreased—warnings

   dvanced breast cancer—indications
A ntacids prior to taking the oral agent
   ssess CBC and hold if WBC< 3500 or platelet count < 100,000

M echanical birth control—for premenopausal women

I ncrease fluid intake to 2-3 per day
   ron and vitamin supplements as ordered

R **O** utine eye exams

X out crushing, breaking, or
   chewing tablets

S unscreen when in the sun
   tore in a light-resistant container

U ndesirable effects—
   DVT, PE, nausea and
   vomiting

N utritious diet

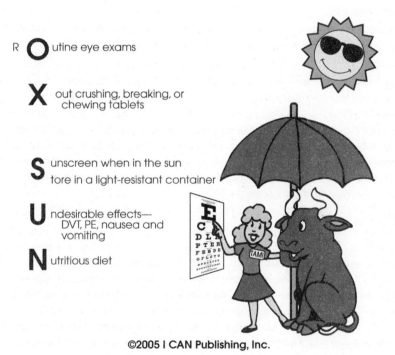

©2005 I CAN Publishing, Inc.

"TAMI" is evaluating the visual acuity of the "OX" since visual acuity may
be affected by the drugs. "TAMI" is protecting the "OX" from the "SUN"
due to photosensitivity. "TAMI OX SUN" will help you remember the agent
tamoxifen.

IMMUNOSUPPRESSIVE AGENT
(Imuran)

Action: Produces immunosuppression by inhibiting purine synthesis in cells.

Indications: Renal tranplants to prevent graft refection, refractory rheumatoid arthritis, refractory ITP, glomerulonephritis, nephrotic syndrome, bone marrow transplant

Warnings: Hypersensitivity. Precautions with severe renal disease or hepatic disease. Elderly.

Undesirable Effects: GI: nausea, vomiting, stomatitis, pancreatitis, hepatotoxicity; HEMA: Leukopenia, thrombocytopenia, anemia, pancytopenia; INTEG: Rash, alopecia; MS: Arthralgia, muscle wasting; MISC: Serum sickness, Raynaud's symptoms.

Other Specific Information: Do not mix with other drugs. **(Imuran)** Leukopenia can result when taken with ACE inhibitors; cotrimoxazole, myelopoiesis. Decreased immune response when taken with vaccines. Decreased action of warfarin. Increased myelosuppression with cyclosporines and antineoplastics. Increased action of azathioprine when taken with allopurinol. Immunosuppression may result when taken with astragalus, echinacea, or melatonin.

Interventions: Assess for infection: increased temperature, WBC; sputum, urine. Assess for rheumatoid arthritis, pain, mobility, ROM; I & O, weight qd, report oliguria; Blood studies: Hgb, WBC, platelets during treatment monthly ; if leukocytes are <3000/mm^3 or platelets <100,000/mm^3, drug should be discontinued. Monitor for hepatotoxicity such as dark urine, jaundice, itching, light-colored stools, increased LFTs; drug should be discontinued. Monitor LFTs: alk phosphatase, AST, ALT, bilirubin. Assess for arthritis: pain; location, ROM, swelling, before and during treatment. All medications po if possible, avoiding IM injections, since bleeding may occur. Administer po with meals to reduce GI upset. For IV route, prepare in biologic cabinet using gown, gloves, mask.

Education: Educate client to take as prescribed, do not miss any dose. If dose is missed on qd regimen, skip dose; if on multiple dosing / day, take as soon as remembered. Therapeutic response may take 3–4 mo. In rheumatoid arthritis; to continue with prescribed exercise, rest, other medication. Report rash, fever, diarrhea that is severe, chills, sore throat, fatigue, due to the fact that serious infections may occur. Instruct client to use contraceptive measures during treatment and for 12 wks after finishing treatment. Avoid vaccinations. Reduce risk of infection by avoiding crowds. Use soft-bristled toothbrush to prevent bleeding.

Evaluation: Absence of graft rejection; immunosuppression in autoimmune disorders.

Drugs: azathioprine (Imuran), tacrolimus (Prograf), cyclosporine (Sandimmune), mycophenolate (CellCept)

IMURAN

I muran, Prograf, Sandimmune, Cellcept—
lessen or prevent immune response

M onitor CBC and liver enzymes

U ses: organ transplantation and autoimmune diseases

R eport fever of 99° farenheit or higher, skin rash, joint pain,
swelling of lymph glands

A dvise to give oral forms with meals

N o liver vaccines

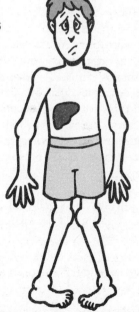

©2005 I CAN Publishing, Inc.

COLONY STIMULATING FACTORS

Action: Erythropoietin is one factor controlling rate of red cell production; drug developed by recombinant DNA technology. Stimulates production of red blood cells. Amino acid polypeptide.

Indications: Anemia resulting from reduced endogenous erythropoietin production, primarily end-stage renal disease; anemia due to AZT treatment in HIV clients; anemia due to chemotherapy.

Warnings: Hypersensitivity to mammalian cell-derived products, or human albumin, uncontrolled hypertension.

Undesirable Effects: Hypertensive encephalopathy, seizures; headache; joint pain

Other Specific Information: Need for increased anticoagulant during hemodialysis

Interventions: Assess renal studies; urinalysis, protein, blood, BUN, creatinine. Blood studies; ferritin, transferrin monthly. Evaluate for rising blood pressure as Hct rises; antihypertensives may be needed. Report drop in urine output less than 50 ml/hour.
Administer only IV or Subcutaneously.

Education: Avoid driving or hazardous activity during beginning of treatment. Monitor Blood pressure. Take iron supplements, vitamin B12, folic acid as directed.

Evaluation: Client will have an increase in the reticulocyte count in 1–6 weeks, Hgb/Hct. Client will have an increased appetite and enhanced sense of well-being.

Drug: epoetin (EPO, Epogen, erythropoietin, Procrit); darbepoetin (Aranesp)

PROCRIT

P roduces erythropoietin

R ed blood cells ↑ (Epogen, Procrit, Aranesp)

O $_2$ ↑ ; decreases fatigue, weakness, SOB

C hemotherapy, cancer

R equires frequent HCTs for dosage adjustment

I V or SQ injection only

T hree times weekly

©2005 I CAN Publishing, Inc.

GRANULOCYTE COLONY-STIMULATING FACTOR

Action: Stimulates proliferation and differentiation of neutrophils.

Indications: To decrease infection in clients receiving antineoplastics that are myelosuppressive; to increase WBC in clients with drug-induced neutropenia; bone marrow transplantation. Investigational uses: Neutropenia in HIV infection.

Warnings: Hypersensitivity to proteins of E. coli. Pregnancy, lactation, cardiac conditions, children, myeloid malignancies.

Undesirable Effects: RESP: Respiratory distress syndrome; CNS: Fever; HEMA: Thrombocytopenia; INTEG: Alopecia, exacerbation of skin conditions; MS: Osteoporosis, skeletal pain; GI: Nausea, vomiting diarrhea, anorexia.

Other Specific Information: Do not use these agents concomitantly with antineoplastics.

Interventions: Assess blood studies: CBC, platelet count before treatment and twice weekly; neutrophil counts may be increased for 2 days after therapy. Assess B/P, respirations, pulse before and during therapy. Assess bone pain, give mild analgesics.

Education: Instruct client on the technique for self-administration: dose, side effects, disposal of containers and needles; provide written instructions.

Evaluation: Absence of infection.

Drugs: fil**grastim** (**Neu**pogen), pegfil**grastim** (**Neu**lasta)

NEUPOGEN

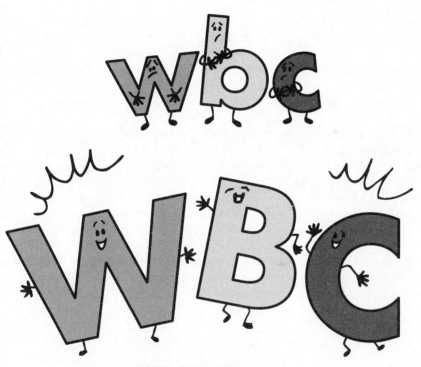

©2005 I CAN Publishing, Inc.

Neupogen is used to increase "new" white blood cells. The "NEU" will assist you in remembering this drug category.

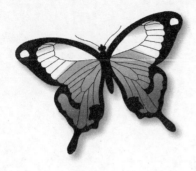

We are all on the way up the mountain and we need each others' help.

Jon Kabat-Zinn

Anti-inflammatory Agents

Editors' Note: *While we have made every effort to include the most up-to-date information regarding these agents, several of these medications were still under investigation for possible increased risk factors at the time of publication.*

—*Loretta and Sylvia*

NONSTEROIDAL ANTI-INFLAMMATORY DRUGS (NSAIDs)

Action: Inhibits prostaglandin synthesis; resulting in analgesic, anti-inflammatory, and antipyretic activities.

Indications: To reduce fever and inflammatory process. Musculoskeletal disorders (e.g., rheumatoid arthritis and osteoarthritis); analgesic for mild to moderate pain.

Warnings: Do NOT give if client is allergic to salicylates or NSAIDs, renal or hepatic disease, asthma, peptic ulcer, bleeding disorders, systemic lupus erythematosus (SLE). Caution with the elderly.

Undesirable Effects: Refer to next page.

Other Specific Information: ↑ the risk of bleeding with oral anticoagulants. ↑ effects of lithium. ↓ effect of loop diuretics; ↓ antihypertensive effects of beta blockers.

Interventions: Monitor CBC, renal and liver function tests. Observe client for bleeding. (Refer to education.)

Education: Instruct client to take with meals. Avoid alcohol and consult with provider about other meds. Advise not to take aspirin or acetaminophen when taking an NSAID. No driving or activities requiring motor response until certain there is no dizziness. Inform dentist and other providers of drug therapy. Discontinue these meds 5 to 7 days before any major procedure or surgery. Report if temperature does not subside, bleeding occurs, or inflammation does not decrease. Periodic eye exams for long-term therapy.

Evaluation: Client will have pain relief, decreased temperature, and improved mobility without undesirable effects from drugs.

Drugs: diclofenac (Voltaren); diflunisal (Dolobid); etodolac (Lodine); fenoprofen (Nalfon); flurbiprofen (Ansaid); ibuprofen (Advil, Medipren, Motrin, Nuprin); indomethacin (Indocin); ketoprofen (Orudis, Oruvail); ketorolac (Toradol); meclofenamate (Meclomen); nabumetone (Relafen); naproxen (Aleve, Anaprox, Naprosyn); oxaprozin (Daypro); piroxicam (Feldene); sulindac (Clinoril); tolmetin (Tolectin)

NSAIDs

N o alcohol

S E: "BIRTH"—see below

A spirin sensitivity—do not give

I nhibits prostaglandins

D o take with food

S top 5–7 days before surgery

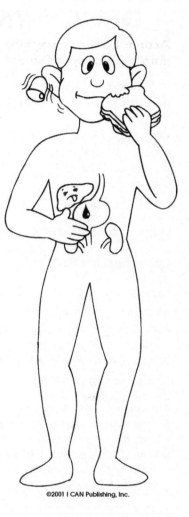

©2001 I CAN Publishing, Inc.

Some side effects include **B**one marrow depression, **I**ncreased GI distress, **R**enal toxicity, **T**innitus and **H**epatotoxicity. Just think that NSAIDs can cause the "death" of inflammation, pain and fever, but the "birth" of undesirable effects.

NONSTEROIDAL ANTI-INFLAMMATORY DRUGS: COX$_2$ INHIBITORS

Action: Inhibition of prostaglandin synthesis, primarily through inhibition of cyclooxygenase-2 (COX$_2$). This results in anti-inflammatory, analgesic, and antipyretic activities.

Indications: Osteoarthritis, rheumatoid arthritis, acute pain in adults.

Warnings: Hypersensitivity; allergic-type reactions to sulfonamides; asthma; urticaria, or allergic-type reaction after taking aspirin or other NSAIDs. GI ulceration, bleeding, or perforation; renal/hepatic; disease; anemia; fluid retention, hypertension, or heart failure; pregnancy/lactation. Bextra can cause Steven-Johnson type reaction.

Undesirable Effects: Refer to next page.

Other Specific Information: Ace Inhibitors and furosemide given concurrently with these drugs may have ↓ effects. Aspirin may result in ↑ rate of GI ulcertaion. Fluconazole may ↑ celebrex levels. Lithium levels may ↑ when given with celebrex. Warfarin may have ↑ risk of bleeding with celebrex predominantly in the elderly.

Interventions: Monitor CBC, liver/renal function tests, and for signs and symptoms of GI bleeding.

Education: Instruct to take with food or meals. Educate client regarding the importance of reporting any signs of GI bleeding or ulceration, skin rash, weight gain or edema, tinnitus, headache, blurred vision, fever, or chills to the health care provider. If visual or CNS disturbances occur, discuss safety measures. Review comfort measures to decrease pain and inflammation (i.e., positioning, warmth, rest, etc.). (Refer to "**NSAIDs**".)

Evaluation: Client will have pain relief, decreased temperature, or improved mobility without undesirable effects.

Drugs: celecoxib (Celebrex); valdecoxib (Bextra)

COX$_2$ INHIBITORS

N o alcohol

S E: "BIRTH"—see below

A spirin sensitivity—do not give

I nhibits COX$_2$ enzyme

D o take with food

S top 5–7 days before surgery

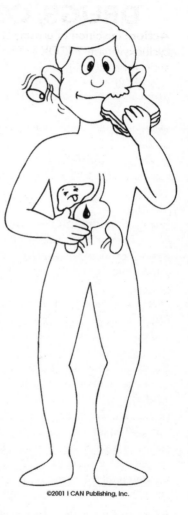

©2001 I CAN Publishing, Inc.

Some side effects include **B**one marrow depression, **I**ncreased GI distress, **R**enal toxicity, **T**innitus and **H**epatotoxicity. Just think that NSAIDs can cause the "death" of inflammation, pain and fever, but the "birth" of undesirable effects.

ANTIGOUT: ALLOPURINOL (ZYLOPRIM)

Action: Reduces production of uric acid by inhibiting xanthine oxidase.

Indications: Gout, recurrent calcium oxalate stones, secondary hyperuricemia which may occur during treatment of leukemia and tumors.

Warnings: Hypersensitivity, renal disease, hepatic disorder.

Undesirable Effects: Anorexia, nausea, vomiting, diarrhea, stomatitis; dizziness, headache; rash, pruritus; metallic taste; retinopathy; bone marrow depression.

Other Specific Information: Alcohol and antacids ↓ effectiveness. Amoxicillin or ampicillin may ↑ incidence of skin rash. Thiazide diuretics ↑ the risk of reactions and ↓ effect. ↑ effect of warfarin, phenytoin, theophylline, anticancer drugs, and ACE inhibitors.

Interventions: Monitor renal and liver functions (*i.e., BUN, serum creatinine, ALP, AST, and ALT*), serum uric acid levels, and CBC prior to initiating therapy, and periodically during therapy. (Refer to Education.)

Education: Increase fluids. May take 1 or more weeks for full therapeutic response. Administer drug following meals; encourage fluid intake (3000 ml/day); monitor intake and output (urinary output should be at least 2000 ml/day). Low purine food intake. Advise to avoid alcohol, caffeine, and large doses of vitamin C. Contact provider if any undesirable effects occur. Recommend a yearly eye examination since visual changes may occur from prolonged use of allopurinol. Driving or activities requiring alertness should be avoided until the response to the medication has been determined.

Evaluation: Client will experience a decrease in joint tenderness, swelling, redness, and fewer acute gout attacks.

Drug: allopurinol (Zyloprim)

GOUT

G ulp 10–12 glasses (8 oz.) of fluid daily
I distress—undesirable effect

O utput and input—monitor closely

U ric acid production decreased
se no alcohol

T ake after meals

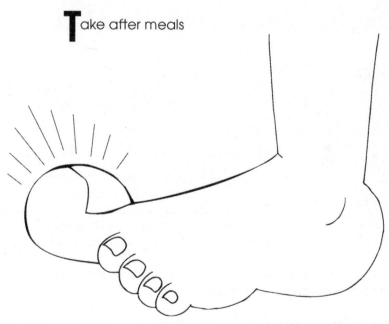

©2001 I CAN Publishing, Inc.

COLCHICINE

Action: Decreases leukocyte motility, phagocytosis, lactic acid production, resulting in decreased urate crystal deposits, inflammatory process.

Indications: Antigout during an initial or acute exacerbation. This may arrest the progression of neurological disability in multiple sclerosis.

Warnings: Severe gastrointestinal, renal, hepatic, or cardiac disorders; blood dyscrasias.

Undesirable Effects: Oliguria, anemias, hypersensitivity, nausea, vomiting, anorexia, diarrhea, cramps.

Other Specific Information: NSAIDs may increase risk of GI distress and anemias. Decrease action of B12.

Interventions: Monitor intake and output. Monitor CBC every 3 months. Evaluate for signs of toxicity including: weakness, abdominal pain, and nausea and vomiting, diarrhea. Discontinue if client experiences weakness, abdominal pain, nausea, vomiting, diarrhea.

Education: Recommend taking with food. Only taken PO or slow IVP (2–5 minutes); never mix with D5W. Avoid any OTC preparation containing alcohol. Report pain, rash, sore throat, bleeding, and/or weakness to the provider of care.

Evaluation: The client will have a decrease stone formation exemplified on x-ray and decrease in the pain in the kidney and/or joints.

Drugs: colchicine

COLCHICINE

A lcohol is out

C uts down on effects of B 12 supplements

U ndesirable effects—oliguria, anemia, nausea, vomiting, anorexia, diarrhea

T ake with food

E xacerbation—gout

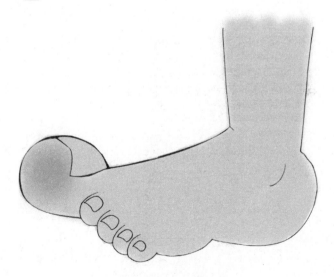

©2004 I CAN Publishing, Inc.

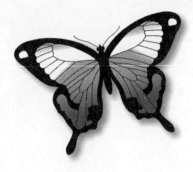

For myself I am an optimist—it does not seem to be much use being anything else.

Sir Winston Churchill

Gastrointestinal Agents

ANTACIDS

Action: Neutralizes gastric acid; decreases pepsin activity.

Indications: Hyperacidity, peptic ulcer, reflux esophagitis.

Warnings: Hypersensitivity to aluminum products, hypophosphatemia, renal failure, obstructive bowel disease, CHF or HTN (Na Citrate). In renal failure, avoid products containing magnesium.

Undesirable Effects: Constipation (Aluminum), diarrhea (Magnesium). Hypercalcemia (in calcium-based antacids); hypermagnesemia (magnesium-calcium containing antacids); hypophosphatemia (long term, aluminum-containing antacids); systemic alkalosis, sodium overload, and rebound acid production (sodium preparation). Renal calculi; all may accumulate in clients with renal failure.

Other Specific Information: Bind, inactivate and / or decrease the absorption of many drugs (too numerous to include total list in this book). Of significant importance is the ↓ in absorption of antibiotics, digoxin, isoniazid, phenothiazine, phenytoin, quinidine.

Interventions: Monitor urinary pH, calcium, electrolytes, and phosphate levels. Record amount and consistency of stools. Clients on low - sodium diets should evaluate sodium content of antacids. (Refer to education)

Education: Instruct to shake suspension well before taking, follow with water. Take 1-3 hours after meals. Do not take within 1-2 hours of other medications. Do not take within 1-2 hours of eating fiber-rich foods. Do not combine with other antacids, calcium supplements (if using calcium-based antacid), or large amounts of caffeine or alcohol. Take calcium carbonate with large amounts of water or orange juice. Advise client to avoid foods or liquids that can cause gastric irritation.

Evaluation: Client will experience relief of heartburn or be absent of pain with no undesirable effects.

Drugs: *Aluminum-based agents*: ALternaGel; Amphogel. ***Magnesium-based agents:*** Milk of Magnesia. ***Aluminum and Magnesium:*** Gaviscon; Maalox; Mylanta; Riopan, Riopan Plus. ***Calcium-based agents:*** Titrilac; Citracal; Tums.

AUNT ACID'S FAMILY

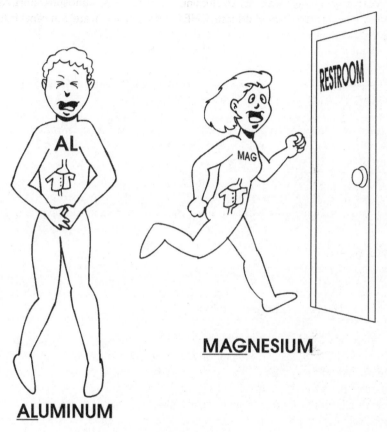

©2001 I CAN Publishing, Inc.

Mag and Al have a history of an ulcer. While the ant-acids, may help in coating their stomachs, they may also experience undesirable effects. **Al's** problem is constipation. **Mag** has a problem with diarrhea.

ANTI-ULCER MEDICATIONS: H$_2$ HISTAMINE ANTAGONISTS

Action: Reduces gastric acid secretions; prevents histamine-induced acid release by competing with histamine for H$_2$ receptors in the stomach.

Indications: Hypersecretion of stomach acids, gastroesophageal reflux, short-term treatment of duodenal ulcers, long-term prophylaxis of duodenal ulcer, prevention of upper GI bleed in critically ill clients.

Warnings: Hypersensitivity; caution with administering cimetidine in clients > 50 years old with renal or liver failure.

Undesirable Effects: Confusion, headache; nausea, diarrhea or consipation; depression; rash; blurred vision. Hepatic/renal toxicity—more profound with cimetidine. Blood dyscrasias are rarely seen.

Other Specific Information: Cimetidine ↑ serum concentrations of many drugs by inhibiting liver P450 enzymes: oral anticoagulants, theophylline, lidocaine, phenytoin, benzodiazipines, nephedipine, propranolol, procainamide. ↓ absorption of ketoconazole. ↓ absorption with antacids.

Interventions: Monitor GI discomfort. Periodic evaluation of blood counts, gastric acid secretion tests, and renal and hepatic function tests. Be alert that the elderly need a decrease in the drug dosage.

Education: Avoid antacids for 1 hour before taking drug. Advise to take with meals. Take Zantac, Pepcid, or Axid at 6pm for better suppression of nocturnal acid secretion. To assist in ↓ acid reflux, advise client to elevate the head of the bed with 6 inch blocks during sleep; wear loose clothing; no meal intake 2 hours prior to hs; eliminate caffeine, alcohol, harsh spices, chocolate, peppermint from diet; stop smoking; no ASA or NSAIDS. Notify provider of blood in emesis or stool or an increase in the abdominal pain.

Evaluation: Peptic ulcer disease eradicated in 4–8 weeks. GERD eradicated in 6–12 weeks. Client will be free of discomfort with no undesirable effects from the medication.

Drugs: (*These drugs end in "dine".*) cimeti**dine** (Tagamet); famoti**dine** (Pepcid); nizati**dine** (Axid); raniti**dine** (Zantac)

NO WINE JUST DINE

D on't take with antacids

I nform provider of bleeding

N o smoking, alcolhol or NSAIDs

E levate head of bed

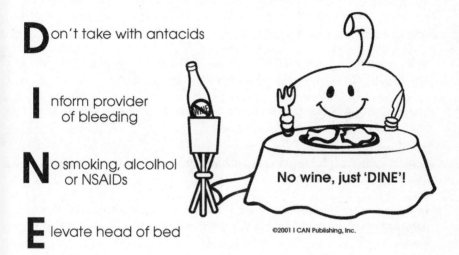

No wine, just 'DINE'!

©2001 I CAN Publishing, Inc.

CIMETI**DINE**
FAMOTI**DINE**
NIZATI**DINE**
RANITI**DINE**

CHOLINERGIC BLOCKERS (ANTICHOLINERGICS)

Action: Blocks cholinergic receptor sites so response to acetylcholine is decreased.

Indications: Bradycardia and heart block; gastrointestinal disorders related to increased motility and secretion (peptic ulcers, diverticulitis, ulcerative colitis); urinary spasms; Parkinson's disease (may also be used to treat extrapyramidal symptoms associated with administration of Thorazine); dilates pupils of the eye. Preoperatively to decrease secretions and vagal stimulation.

Warnings: Glaucoma, myasthenia gravis, obstructive GI disorders, prostatic hypertrophy, children less than 3 years of age; elderly.

Undesirable Effects: Dilated pupils, distended bladder, dry mucous membranes, constipation, increased heart rate.

Other Specific Information: ↑ anticholinergic effect with antidepressants, MAOIs, and phenothiazines.

Interventions: Monitor VS, report ↑ HR; monitor for constipation, oliguria. Atropine could result in CNS stimulation (confusion, excitement), or drowsiness.

Education: Instruct to take 30 minutes before meals; eat foods high in fiber and drink plenty of fluids. Avoid OTC antihistamines. Instruct client not to drive a motor vehicle or participate in activities requiring alertness. Advise to use hard candy, ice chips, etc. for dry mouth. Recommend artificial tears.

Evaluation: The client will experience symptomatic relief with no undesirable effects.

Drugs: atropine (Isopto Atropine); benztropine mesylate (Cogentin); dicyclomine (Bentyl); glycopyrrolate (Robinul); procyclidine (Kemadrin); propantheline (Pro-Banthine); scopolamine (Isopto Hyoscine, Transderm-Scop); trihexyphenidyl (Artane)

ANTICHOLINERGICS

Can't pee
Can't see
Can't spit
Can't shit

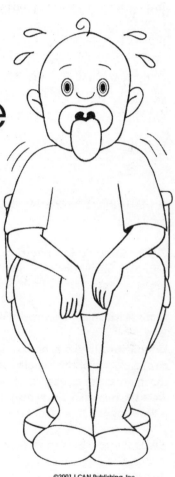

©2001 I CAN Publishing, Inc.

PROTON PUMP INHIBITOR

Action: Suppresses the final step in gastric acid production by forming a covalent bond to two sites of the (H^+, K^+)-ATPase enzyme system at the surface of the gastric parietal cell. This results in an increase in the gastric pH, reducing gastric acid production.

Indications: Short-term treatment of erosive esophagitis associated with gastroesophageal reflux disease (GERD). Omeprazole—Long-term treatment of active duodenal ulcer. Maintenance of erosive esophagitis. Treatment of H. Pylori (with amoxicillin), active benign gastric ulcers. Prevacid and Protonix are available in IV. May see off-label use for stress ulcer prophylaxis and GI bleed. Prevacid IV must be administered with a filter. Both may be given as a continuous infusion.

Warnings: Hypersensitivity; pregnancy/lactation; safety and efficacy of pantoprazole for maintenance therapy beyond 16 weeks have not been established.

Undesirable Effects: Headache, dizziness, diarrhea, abdominal discomfort, flatulence.

Other Specific Information: May ↑ concentration of oral anticoagulants, diazepam, phenytoin when administered with omeprazole. No clinically relevant interactions with pantoprazole.

Interventions: Monitor for GI symptoms or headache.

Education: Take omeprazole before meals; pantoprazole once or twice a day. Instruct client to report headache to the provider of care. Emphasize the importance of only remaining on the pantoprazole for a maximum of 16 weeks. Omeprazole may need to be taken for up to 8 wks. Regular medical follow-ups are important for evaluation.

Evaluation: Client should experience relief of gastrointestinal symptoms.

Drugs: omeprazole (Prilosec); pantoprazole (Protonix), lansoprazole (Prevacid), rabeprazole (Aciphen), esomeprazole (Nexium)

PROTON PUMP INHIBITOR

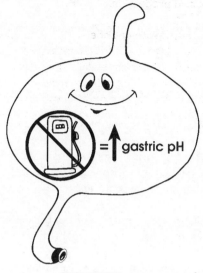

=↑ gastric pH

©2001 I CAN Publishing, Inc.

P rilosec—only p. o.

U E: headache, G I disturbances

M aximum of 16 weeks for Protonix

P rotonix—can be given IV
prevacid

PEPSIN INHIBITOR: CARAFATE

Action: Forms a protective covering on the ulcer surface, protecting ulcer from acid, bile salts, and pepsin; also inhibits pepsin activity in gastric juices.

Indications: Short-term treatment of duodenal ulcers (up to 8 weeks); NSAID or aspirin induced GI symptoms; prevention of stress ulcers in critically ill clients.

Warnings: Hypersensitivity, renal failure, pregnancy, lactation.

Undesirable Effects: Dizziness, nausea, constipation.

Other Specific Information: ↓ effectiveness of ciprofloxacin, norfloxacin, penicillamine, phenytoin. Altered absorption with antacids. Risk of aluminum toxicity with aluminum-containing antacids.

Interventions: Monitor the characteristics of the abdominal pain, renal function, fluid and electrolytes, and gastric pH (>5 is desired).

Education: Instruct to administer drug on an empty stomach. Administer antacids 30 minutes before or after sucralfate. Allow 1 to 2 hours between sucralfate and other medications; sucralfate binds with certain drugs, reducing the effect of the drugs. Instruct to take drug as ordered. It usually takes 4–8 weeks for optimal ulcer healing. Recommend fluid, fiber, and exercise to decrease constipation. Recommend no smoking and no foods and liquids that can cause gastric distress. Report pain or vomiting of blood.

Evaluation: Client will be free of pain and will experience no undesirable effects of med.

Drug: sucralfate (Carafate)

CARA

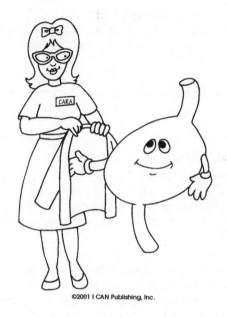

©2001 I CAN Publishing, Inc.

C onstipation—undesirable effect

A dminister on an empty stomach

R isk of aluminum toxicity with aluminum antacids

A dminister antacids 30 min. before or after med.

Cara is holding the coat that goes on the stomach. Carafate will form a protective coating on the ulcer surface. It protects against pepsin and acid.

ANTIDIARRHEAL: LOMOTIL

Action: Inhibits gastric motility.

Indications: Acute diarrhea.

Warnings: Child <2; pregnancy; elderly; antibiotic associated colitis or ulcerative colitis; hepatic/renal disease; glaucoma; electrolyte imbalance. Do not use if client has C. diff.

Undesirable Effects: Drowsiness, dizziness, constipation, dry mouth, blurred vision, urinary retention.

Other Specific Information: Alcohol, MAO inhibitors, antihistamines, narcotics, and sedative-hypnotics may interact with drugs.

Interventions: During the history, determine cause of diarrhea. Monitor stools for frequency and consistency, bowel sounds, I & O, vital signs, and electrolytes. Evaluate hydration especially in the very young and very old. Report if client has a narcotic drug history.

Education: Encourage clear liquids. Avoid OTC drugs and alcohol. Avoid activities requiring alertness, motor activities, until response to drug is evaluated. Notify provider for diarrhea that persists longer than 2 days, high fever, blood in stool, or acute abdominal pain. Advise client that these drugs can be habit forming, so only take the prescribed dose.

Evaluation: Client will have no diarrhea.

Drugs: (*C-V Controlled Substance*) diphenoxylate with atropine (Logen, Lomanate, Lomotil, Lonox)

ANTIDIARRHEALS

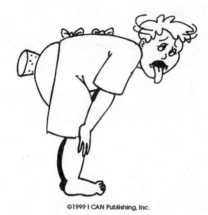

©1999 I CAN Publishing, Inc.

D rowsiness, dizziness, dry mouth, dehydration

I nhibits gastric mobility

A lcohol is OUT!

R eport if there is a narcotic drug history

R esponse of drug determined prior to driving

H abit forming—only take prescribed dose

E lectrolytes—monitor with severe diarrhea;
    encourage clear liquids

A ssess frequency of bowel movements; bowel sounds

BULK FORMING: METAMUCIL

Action: Bulk-forming laxative by drawing water.

Indications: Chronic constipation.

Warnings: Hypersensitivity, abdominal discomfort, fecal impaction, intestinal obstruction.

Undesirable Effects: Anorexia, cramps, nausea, vomiting, diarrhea, intestinal obstruction if not taken with adequate water.

Other Specific Information: ↓ absorption of aspirin, oral anticoagulant, digoxin, nitrofurantoin.

Interventions: Monitor VS, I & O, signs of fluid and electrolyte imbalance, and bowel sounds. Assess cause of constipation.

Education: Instruct to mix the drug in 8-10 oz. of water, stir, and drink immediately. Do not swallow in dry form. Follow drug with 1 extra glass of water. Instruct client to drink a minimum of eight 8 oz. glasses of water per day and to increase foods high in fiber. Review the nonpharmacologic methods for decreasing constipation. Review the importance of not becoming a habitual user of laxatives.

Evaluation: Client will have regular bowel movements with no constipation.

Drug: psyllium (Metamucil)

SILLY PSYLLIUM

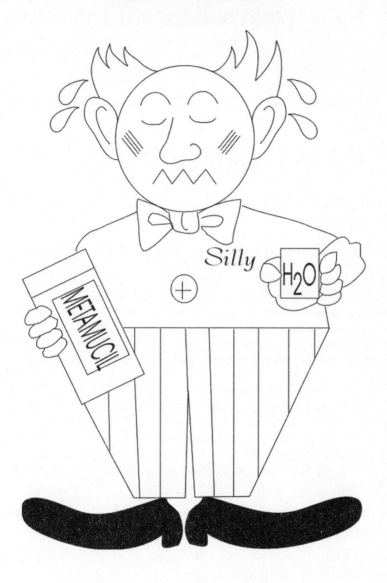

Silly got his name by taking psyllium (Metamucil) with a jigger of water instead of a BIG glass of water. Now he's sweating because this bulk-forming laxative that expands has bulked his bow tie instead of his stool.

LAXATIVES: STIMULANT/EMOLLIENT

Action: Stimulant: Increases peristalsis by direct effect on colonic smooth musculature. Laxative effect is a result of the promotion of fluid and ion accumulation in the colon.
Emollient: Softens stools by increasing the water and fat penetration in the intestines.

Indications: Constipation, Evacuation of colon for bowel examination, rectal, and/or elective colon surgery. Stool softener; facilitates passage of stools. Prevention of constipation in cardiac/post surgical procedures.

Warnings: Hypersensitivity, fecal impactions, intestinal/biliary obstruction, nausea and vomiting, acute hepatitis, appendicitis, and/or acute surgical abdomen.

Undesirable Effects: Nausea, anorexia, cramping, and/or diarrhea.

Other Specific Information: Stimulant: Gastric irritation if taken with antacids, H2-blockers, and gastric proton pump inhibitors, and milk.
Emollient: If taken with mineral oil, may result in toxicity.

Interventions: Monitor intake and output, bowel sounds, and serum electrolytes, and/or abdominal pain and cramping.

Education: *Emollients:* May take up to 3 days to soften stools. Take tablets whole. Do not take for long term therapy.
Both: Report cramping, weakness, dizziness, and an increase in being thirsty. Inform provider if constipation is unrelieved or symptoms of electrolyte imbalance occur: muscle cramps, pain, weakness, dizziness, excessive thirst. Teach family and client that normal bowel movements do not always occur daily.

Evaluation: Client will have regular bowel movements with no constipation or straining.

Drug: *Stimulant:* bisacodyl (Carter's Little Pills, Dulcolax, Dacodyl, Feen-a-mint, Fleet Laxative, Therelax)
Emollient: docusate calcium (Surfax, DC Softgels); docusate sodium (Colace, Ex-Lax, Modane, Silace)

COLACE

Cause of constipation (fluids, bulks, decrease exercise)

Dulc**O**lax—most common drug producing bowel stimulation

F **L**uid—increase intake

T **A**ste bitter; give in milk or juice to mask

Cardiac/surgical procedures—to minimize straining

Electrolytes

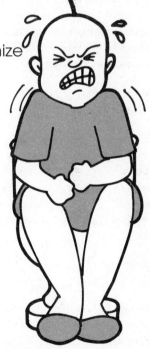

©2005 I CAN Publishing, Inc.

ANTIEMETIC:
Torecan

Action: Acts centrally by blocking chemoreceptor trigger zone This will in turn act on the vomiting center.

Indications: Nausea and Vomiting

Warnings: Hypersensitivity to phenothiazines, coma, seizures, encephalopathy, bone marrow depression.

Other Specific Information: Decreases the effect of thiethylperazine: barbituates, antacids. Increases the anticholinergic action: anticholinergics, antiparkinson drugs, and antidepressants.

Interventions: Assess the vital signs and blood pressure. Assess client with cardiac disease for neuroleptic malignant syndrome: dyspnea, fever, seizures, diaphoresis, fatigue, and tachycardia. Assess respiratory status before, during, and after administration. Respiratory distress may occur in the older client. If administered IM, client should remain recumbent 1 hour after the injection.

Education: Instruct client to avoid hazardous activities or activities that require alertness.

Staff Education: Do not confuse Torecan with Toradol.

Evaluation: The client will experience an absence of nausea and vomiting.

Drug: thiethylperazine (Norzine, Torecan)

"ANTI EM"

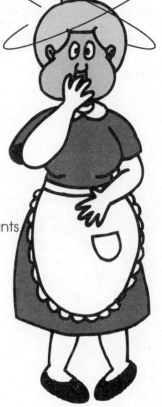

A ssess bowel sounds

N o alcohol or other CNS depressants

T ake prophylactically

I nteracts with medications

E valuate for changes (hypovolemia, hypotension, dry mouth, oliguria, dry eyes)

M onitor for mental changes

©2005 I CAN Publishing, Inc.

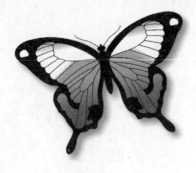

We make a living by what we get, we make a life by what we give.

Sir Winston Churchill

Endocrine Agents

CORTICOSTEROIDS

Action: Synthesized by adrenal cortex. Exhibits antiinflammatory properties; suppresses the normal immune response. Increases carbohydrate, fat, and protein metabolism.

Indications: Antiinflammatory; immunosuppressant; dermatological disorders; replacement in adrenal cortical insufficiency.

Warnings: Hypersensitivity; PUD; tuberculosis, fungal infections or any suspected infection; HIV; blood clotting disorders; renal hepatic impairment; cardiac disease, congestive heart failure, hypertension; diabetes mellitus; geriatric client, and postmenopausal women.

Undesirable Effects: Undesirable effects rarely seen with short-term high dose or replacement therapy. "**CUSHING**" will help you in recalling effects that may occur with long-term use. Cushing-like symptoms (moon-face, excess fat deposits at trunk, wasting of arms and legs—refer to Cushy Carl on next page). To assist you in remembering that the sodium ↑, potassium ↓, glucose ↑, and calcium levels ↓, refer to next page.

Other specific information: ↑ risk of hypokalemia with diuretics, amphotericin B, ticarcillin. ↓ effects of antidiabetics, vaccines, potassium supplements. May ↑ digoxin toxicity (due to hypokalemia).

Interventions: Monitor VS, BP, weight, blood glucose, electrolytes, EKG, and TB skin test results.

Education: Instruct to administer oral drugs with food or milk early in the morning; withdraw medication slowly. Follow-up visits and lab tests are essential. Avoid infection. Taper off gradually under medical supervision. Report visual disturbance or severe GI distress, sudden weight gain, swelling, sore throat, fever, or signs of infection. Wounds may heal slowly. Avoid crowds and known infection. Do not receive vaccination. Don't take aspirin or any medication without consulting provider. Discuss a diet low in sodium, high in vitamin D, protein and potsassium. Inform provider of therapy. Don't overuse. For topical applications, apply after shower. Do not cover. Avoid sun light on treated area. Recommend wearing a medical alert tag.

Evaluation: The client will experience an improvement in the underlying condition for which the corticosteroids were given and will have no undesirable effects.

Drugs: *(Many of these end in "one")* **Topical:** alclometas**one** (Acolvate); amcinonide (Cyclocort); betametha**sone** (Celestone, Diprosone, Uticort, Valisone—O, IV, IL, IA); clobetasol (Temovate); cortis**one** (Cortone—O); desoride (Tridesilone); desoximetas**one** (Topicort); dexamethas**one** (Decadron—O, IM, IV, OP, IN, IH); fluocino**lone** (Synalar, Synemol); flurandrenolide (Cordran); fluticasone (Cutivate, Flonase—IN); halcinonide (Halog); halobetasol (Ultravate); hydrocortis**one** (Cort-Dome, Cortef, Hydrocortone, Solu-Cortef—O, IM, IV, SubQ, R); mometasone (Elocon); prednicarbate (Dermatop); *Inhalation, intranasal:* beclomethas**one** (Beclovent, Vanceril, Beconase, Vancenase); budesonide (Rhinocort—IN only); flunisolide (Aerobid, Nasalide); triamcinol**one** (Azmacort, Kenalog, Nasacort—O); **Oral:** fludrocortis**one** (Florinef); methylprednisol**one** (Medrol, Solu-Medrol—IM, IV); prednisol**one** (Delta-Cortef, Hydeltra, Hydeltrasol —IM, IV, IL, IA); prednis**one** (Deltasone, Meticorten, Orasone). **Ophthalmic:** fluorometh**olone** (FML); nmexol**one** (Vexol).

Key: Intraarticular = IA, Inhalation = IH, Intralesional = IL, Intramuscular = IM, Intranasal = IN, Intravenous = IV, Oral = O, Ophthalmic = OP, Rectal = R, Subcutaneous = SubQ

CUSHY CARL

C ushing-like symptoms

b **U** ffalo hump

S odium
sweating

H eadache
hyperglycemia

I ncrease in BP, HR, appetite

N ot healing quickly

G I upset

Some People Get Cold

S odium↑

Potassium↓

Glucose↑

Calcium↓

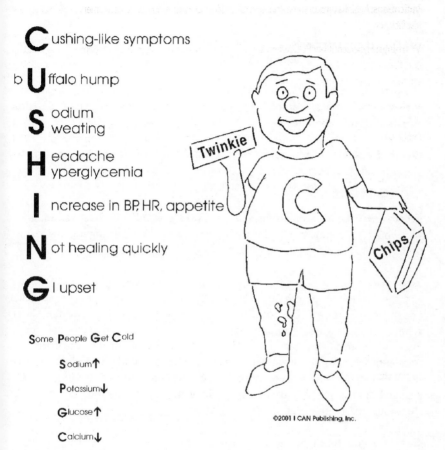

©2001 I CAN Publishing, Inc.

Cushy Carl has taken cortisone for a long time and illustrates some of the undesirable effects with his moon face, buffalo hump, and delay in wound healing (sore on leg). Twinkies and chips are a no-no! "**Some People Get Cold**" is a way to help you remember some lab changes that can occur with "**Cushy Carl**". The labs would be opposite for Addison's Disease.

THYROID PREPARATIONS

Action: Increases the metabolic rate, oxygen consumption, and body growth.

Indications: Hypothyroidism, myxedema, cretinism.

Warnings: Thyrotoxicosis, MI, cardiovascular disease, hypertension, renal disease. Caution in the elderly client.

Undesirable Effects: Vomiting, diarrhea, weight loss; tachycardia, palpitations, angina; nervousness, tremors, irritability, insomnia; menstrual irregularities, sweating, heat intolerance.

Other Specific Information : ↓ effects of antidiabetic agents and digtialis preparation. ↑ effects of oral anticoagulants, sympathomimetics, and antidepressants. ↓ absorption with cholestyramine, colestipol.

Interventions: Monitor serum T_3, T_4, and TSH levels. Obtain baseline vital signs and weight to compare with future assessments. If converting levothyroxine po to IV while in hospital, the IV dose should be 1/2 the oral dose!

Education: Advise client that within 3–4 days there should be improvement and the maximum effect is usually in 4–6 weeks. Teach to take a single daily dose before breakfast. Do not discontinue without consulting provider. Keep scheduled appointments to have periodic blood tests and medical evaluation. Instruct to report signs and symptoms of hypothyroidism (T, P, and BP are usually decreased) and hyperthyroidism (tachycardia and palpitations usually occur). Instruct how to take pulse and to hold medication if > 100. Do not change brands since they are not bioequivalent. Instruct client to have a medic alert tag, card, or bracelet in case of emergency.

Evaluation: The client will be involved in the activities of daily living without becoming tired. Adequate thyroid hormone levels will be attained.

Drugs: levothyroxine T_4 (Eltroxin, Levothroid, Levoxyl, Synthroid); liothyronine T_3 (Cytomel)

MORBID MATILDA

T SH, T_3, T_4—monitor

H ypo/hyperthyroidism—monitor

R eview how to take a pulse

O bserve clinical improvement
      in 3—4 days

I ncrease metabolic rate—action

©2001 I CAN Publishing, Inc.

D o NOT change brands of drug

Synthroid gives Morbid Matilda a boost so she will be less tired.

ANTITHYROID

Action: Inhibits the synthesis of thyroid hormones.

Indications: Hyperthyroidism.

Warnings: Hypersensitivity, lactation.

Undesirable effects: Paresthesia, neuritis, drowsiness, vertigo, nausea, vomiting, agranulocytosis, granulocytopenia, thrombocytopenia, bleeding, skin rash.

Other Specific Information: Altered effects of oral anticoagulants. ↑ concentration of digoxin. I^{131} may be ↓ .

Interventions: Regular blood tests to monitor bone marrow depression and bleeding tendencies. Assess for signs and symptoms of a thyroid crisis (thyroid storm). Monitor vital signs (with hyperthyroidism, tachycardia and palpitations usually occur).

Education: Instruct to take the drug with meals; take 3 equal doses at 8-hour intervals around the clock; do not abruptly stop. Foods containing iodine may be restricted such as salt, shellfish, and OTC cough medicines. Report fever, sore throat, unusual bleeding or bruising, headache or general malaise. Advise client that signs and symptoms of hyperthyroidism should be alleviated in 1-3 weeks. Review signs and symptoms of hypothyroidism since it can occur as a result of treatment. Inform medical staff that client is taking this drug due to increase risk of bleeding.

Evaluation: Client will have a decrease in signs of hyperthyroidism with no undesirable effects.

Drugs: methimazole (Tapazole), propylthiouracil (PTU)

GO GETTER GERTRUDE

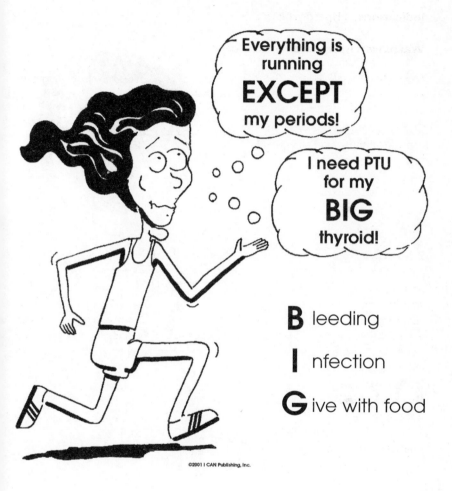

B leeding

I nfection

G ive with food

Gertrude Graves needs some PTU for her "**BIG**" thyroid. These anti-thyroid drugs can cause some problems with bleeding and infection. Taking them with food will decrease GI distress.

HYPOGLYCEMIA

Tremors
achycardia

Irritability

Restless

Excessive hunger

Diaphoresis
epression

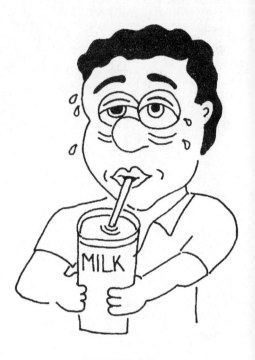

© 2001 I CAN Publishing, Inc.

Hypoglycemia
*(sung to the tune of
"Row, Row, Row Your Boat")*

Hot and dry
Your sugar's high.
Your insulin is what you need.

Cold and clammy
You need some candy,
And milk will help indeed.

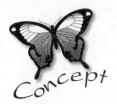

Concept

DIABETES

D iet, weight loss, exercise

I dentification—medical alert bracelet
V only Regular Insulin/Lispro (Humalog)

A void alcohol and other meds

B lood sugar and urine sugar, Hb A_{1c}

E d. about antidiabetic agents

T ranscribe orders—"units" not "u"
herapy decreases signs, not a cure
wo nurses verify dosage administration

E d.—foot care, no smoking, stressors

S igns and symptoms of hyper/hypoglycemia—
     how to do self-monitoring
kin care

©2001 I CAN Publishing, Inc.

ANTIDIABETIC: METFORMIN

Action: Decreases hepatic glucose production and intestinal absorption of glucose; increases peripheral insulin uptake and utilization.

Indications: Non-insulin dependent diabetes.

Warnings: Hypersensitivity; renal/hepatic disease; metabolic acidosis. Clients undergoing radiological studies involving parenteral administration of iodinated contrast materials should be temporarily stopped. Use caution when giving to elderly or malnourished client.

Undesirable Effects: Anorexia, abdominal gas or pain, headache, nausea, vomiting, possible metallic taste; hypoglycemia. *Toxic:* Lactic acidosis.

Other Specific Information: Calcium channel blockers, alcohol, digoxin, vancomycin, furosemide, may ↑ metformin concentration. ↑ risk of hypoglycemia with celery, coriander, dandelion root, garlic, ginseng.

Interventions: Monitor CBC, blood and urine for glucose and ketones, and Hb A_{1c}. Monitor renal function prior to therapy and at least annually to determine normal renal function. Discontinue if the client enters a hypoxic state.

Education: Instruct to take with meals and encourage adequate hydration. Instruct client to discontinue drug and notify provider immediately if experiences unexplained hypoxemia, dehydration, or signs of lactic acidosis (unexplained hyperventilation, muscle aches, fatigue, and lethargy). Notify provider for problems with diarrhea and vomiting. (Refer to "**DIABETES**".)

Evaluation: The client's Hb A_{1c} and serum glucose level will remain within the normal limit, and client will experience no undesirable effects.

Drug: metformin (Glucophage)

METFORMIN

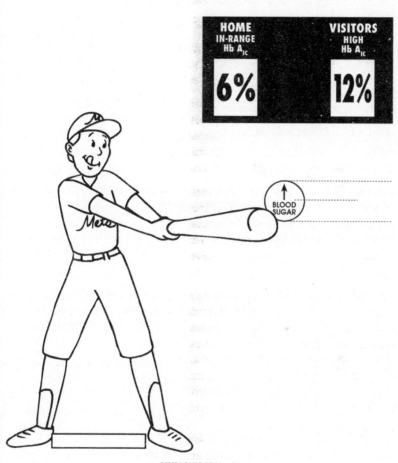

©2001 I CAN Publishing, Inc.

Metformin "The Mets" (glucophage) bats against high blood sugar. He scores the winning home run by decreasing hepatic glucose production and intestinal absorption of glucose, while improving insulin sensitivity. Prior to playing in the big league, he must have a sports physical to check his renal function. A major complication with this medicine is lactic acidosis.

ANTIDIABETIC DRUGS: SULFONYLUREAS

Action: Not fully known. Stimulates insulin release from the pancreatic beta cells and reduces glucose output by the liver. Increases peripheral sensitivity to insulin.

Indications: Non-insulin dependent diabetes Type II (maturity-onset diabetes).

Warning: Allergies to sulfonylureas; Type I insulin dependent diabetes except in conjunction with insulin; diabetes complicated by ketoacidosis; renal/ hepatic disease; cardiac or thyroid disease.

Undesirable Effects: Nausea, vomiting, diarrhea, rash, pruritis, headache, hypoglycemia.

Other Specific Information: ↑ hypoglycemic effect with aspirin, alcohol, anticoagulants, anticonvulsants, sulfonamides, oral contraceptives, MAOIs, and some NSAIDs. ↓ hypoglycemic effect with cortisone, thiazide diuretics, calcium channel blockers, estrogen, phenytoin, thyroid drugs. ↑ risk of hypoglycemia with celery, coriander, dandelion root, garlic, ginseng.

Interventions: Monitor vital signs, BUN, serum creatinine, liver function tests, blood and urine glucose, and Hb A_{1c}. Chlorpropamide is not a desirable choice for the elderly client due to long duration of action. The second-generation agents may be safer for this group of clients with respect to drug interactions. Monitor elderly for hypersensitivity. Drug may accumulate in client with renal insufficiency. (Refer to "**DIABETES**".)

Education: Instruct client to take with food. Review with client that insulin might be necessary instead of an oral antidiabetic medication during a serious infection, stressful time, or surgery. Discuss the importance of eating meals on schedule since missing a meal can result in hypoglycemia. (Refer to "**DIABETES**".)

Evaluation: The client's Hb A_{1c} and serum glucose level will be within the normal range, and the client will be able to safely manage the oral antidiabetic agents.

Drugs: *first generation:* acetohexamide (Dymelor); chlorpropamide (Diabinese); tolazamide (Tolinase); tolbutamide (Orinase); ***second generation:*** glimepiride (Amaryl); glipizide (Glucotrol, Glucotrol XL); glyburide (Diabeta, Glynase PresTab, Micronase)

SULFONYLUREAS

G limepiride lipizide **are better for** **G** randmother

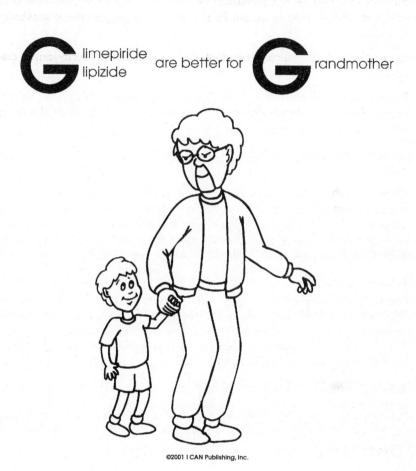

©2001 I CAN Publishing, Inc.

Chlorpropamide is not good for Grandmother (geriatic client) due to its long duration of action. Grandmother has a shorter span to live than her grandchild, so she needs the agent with the shorter duration of action.

INSULIN SENSITIZER: AVANDIA

Action: Stimulates insulin receptor sites to lower serum glucose and improve the action of insulin.

Indication: Monotherapy for Type II diabetes; combination with metformin when diet, exercise, and either agent alone are not effective with Type II diabetes.

Warnings: Hepatic disease, Class III-IV cardiac disease, premenopausal anovulatory women.

Undesirable effects: Headache, hypoglycemia, elevations in liver enzymes, anemia.

Other Specific Information: ↓ effectiveness of oral contraceptives.

Interventions: Monitor liver function tests, serum and urine glucose, and CBC. If client switches from troglitazone, do not start rosiglitazone for 7 days after stopping the troglitazone.

Education: Advise client to take with meals. If dose is missed, it may be taken at the next meal. Do not double dose the next day, if dose is missed for an entire day. Provide educational offerings regarding the disease, dietary control, exercise, avoidance of infection, hygiene, and signs and symptoms of hypo/hyperglycemia. Review the importance of using a barrier contraceptive if taking oral contraceptives.

Evaluation: Client's serum and urine glucose and Hb A_{1c} will remain within the normal range, and client will experience no undesirable effects from the medication.

Drug: rosiglitazone (Avandia), pioglitazone (Actos)

AVANDIA

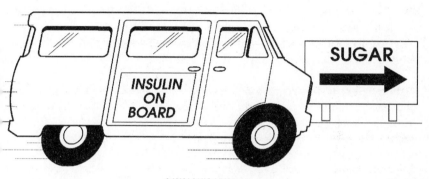

© 2001 I CAN Publishing, Inc.

S igns of anemia, ↑ liver enzymes: UE

U se barrier contraceptives

G lucose urine and serum—monitor

A dminister with meals

R osiglitazone (Avandia)

This van is improving the action of insulin, which helps in the management of diabetes. "**SUGAR**" will assist you with the key points.

INSULIN

Action: Reduces blood sugar level by increasing glucose transport across muscle and fat cell. Promotes conversion of glucose to glycogen.

Indications: Diabetes Mellitus; diabetic ketoacidosis; to lower blood sugar.

Warnings: Pregnancy/lactation.

Undesirable Effects: Hypoglycemia (refer to **"TIRED"**) Tremors, tachycardia, Irritability, Restless, Excessive hunger, Diaphoresis, depression. Rebound hyperglycemia (Somogyi effect); redness, irritation or swelling at injection site; flushing; urticaria; lipodystrophy.

Other Specific Information: ↑ hypoglycemic effect with aspirin, oral anticoagulant, alcohol, beta blockers, oral hypoglycemics, MAOIs, tricyclic antidepressants, tetracycline. ↓ hypoglycemic effect with thiazides, glucocorticoids, oral contraceptives, thyroid drugs, smoking. ↑ risk of hypoglycemia with celery, coriander, dandelion root, garlic, ginseng.

Interventions: Monitor vital signs, blood and urine glucose levels, and Hb A_{1c}. Insulin can be used to manage diabetes in the pregnant woman; however, client must be monitored closely. Dosage is always expressed in USP units. Use syringes calibrated for the particular concentration of insulin administered. Humalog is the fastest acting insulin, acting within 15 minutes; may be given I.V. (Refer to **"DIABETES"**.)

Education: Whenever NPH or Lente is mixed with regular insulin in the same syringe, give it immediately to avoid loss of potency. (Refer to image on page 176 for mixing insulin.) Avoid insulin that changes color or becomes clumped or granular in appearance. Dosage may vary with activities, diet, or stress. Chart and rotate injection sites. Store in refrigerator. (Refer to **"DIABETES"**.)

Evaluation: Blood sugar and Hb A_{1c} will be within normal limits, and client will manage insulin safely.

Drugs: *Rapid-Acting:* Humalog; Regular (Humulin R, Ilentin Regular, Novolin R, Velosulin BR); *Intermediate-Acting:* NPH (Humulin N, Ilentin NPH, Novolin N); Lente (Humulin L, Ilentin L, Novolin L); *Long-Acting:* PZI (Humulin U), Lantus; *Combination Insulins:* NPH and Regular (Humulin 70/30, Novolin 70/30, Humulin 50/50)

PEAK TIMES FOR INSULIN

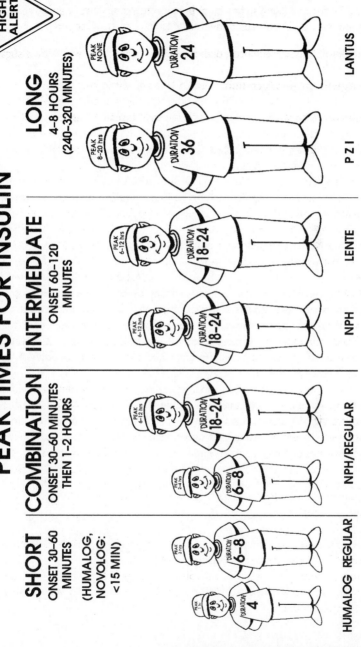

HIGH ALERT

SHORT
ONSET 30–60 MINUTES

(HUMALOG, NOVOLOG: <15 MIN)

COMBINATION
ONSET 30–60 MINUTES THEN 1–2 HOURS

INTERMEDIATE
ONSET 60–120 MINUTES

LONG
4–8 HOURS (240–320 MINUTES)

HUMALOG — PEAK 1 hr — DURATION 4

REGULAR — PEAK 3 hrs — DURATION 6–8

NPH/REGULAR — PEAK 2–4 hrs — DURATION 6–8 ; PEAK 6–12 hrs — DURATION 18–24

NPH — PEAK 6–12 hrs — DURATION 18–24

LENTE — PEAK 6–12 hrs — DURATION 18–24

P Z I — PEAK 8–20 hrs — DURATION 36

LANTUS — PEAK NONE — DURATION 24

Insulins vary in their onset, peak and duration.

INSULIN LISPRO (HUMALOG)

Action: Antidiabetic (pancreatic hormone)

Indications: Rapid-acting insulin used to treat elevated glucose levels in type 1 and type 2 diabetes (usually in addition to intermediate and long-acting insulins, or, with type 2 diabetes, oral hypoglycemic agents).

Warnings: **HIGH ALERT DRUG** Allergy or hypersensitivity.

Undesirable Effects: Urticaria, HYPOGLYCEMIA, rebound hyperglycemia (Somogyi effect), lipodystrophy, itiching, redness, swelling, allergic reactions including ANAPHYLAXIS.

Other Specific Information: Refer to Insulin.

Interventions: *Adults:* 5–10 units up to 15 min. before meals. Use only U-100 insulin syringes to draw up insulin lispro dose. Do not accept insulin orders that contain the abbreviation "U" for units. It has been misread as a zero, which resulted in serious, ten-fold over dose. Clarify any order that contains this abbreviation. Hypoglycemia is most likely to occur 2–4 hours after administration. Assess client for signs and symptoms of hypoglycemia.

Education: Instruct client when mixing insulins to draw insulin lispro into syringe first to avoid contamination of insulin lispro vial. Instruct client and family about signs and symptoms of hyper and hypoglcemia. Instruct client regarding importance of eating meal after receiving medication. Do not wait for an extended period of time to eat. Client may get hypoglycemic.

Staff Education: Do not confuse Humalog with Humulin.

Evalution: Client's blood sugar will remain within the therapeutic range.

Drugs: Insulin lispro (Humalog), Insulin Aspart (Novolog)

LISPRO

HIGH ALERT

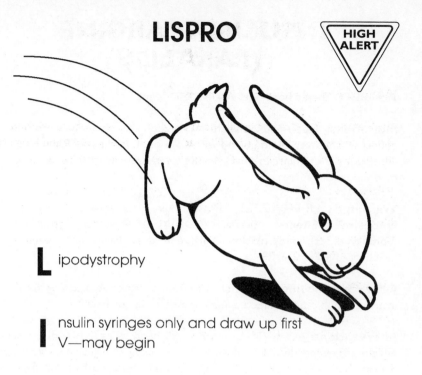

L ipodystrophy

I nsulin syringes only and draw up first
V—may begin

S taff education—don't confuse Humalog
with Humalin

P refilled syringes stable for one week

R apid action, have food nearby

O bserve for hypoglycemic reactions

©2005 I CAN Publishing, Inc.

Hoppy Humalog is quick! He rapidly decreases glucose levels.

INSULIN GLARGINE (LANTUS)

Action: Pancreatic hormone. Antidiabetic agent.

Indications: Type 1 and 2 diabetes. Long-acting insulin with a constant concentration over 24 hours and with no pronounced peak. Provides a continuous level of insulin similar to the steady secretion of insulin provided by the normal pancreas.

Warnings: HIGH ALERT DRUG   Allergy or hypersensitivity.
Undesirable Effects: Urticaria, HYPOGLYCEMIA, rebound hyperglycemia (Somogyi effect), lipodystrophy, itching, redness, swelling, allergic reactions including ANAPHYLAXIS.

Other Specific Information: Lantus insulin cannot be mixed with other insulins; action may be affected in an unpredictable manner.

Interventions: Assess client for signs of hypoglycemia (cool, clammy skin, difficulty concentrating, drowsiness; excessive hunger; headache; irritability; nausea; rapid pulse; shakiness) and hyperglycemia (hot, flushed skin; fruity breath; polyuria; loss of appetite; tiredness; thirsty) throughout therapy.

Education: Usually begin with 10 units at bedtime and titrate according to glucose levels. Use only insulin syringes to draw up dose. Rotate injection sites.

Staff Education: Do not accept insulin orders that contain the abbreviation "U" for "units." It can be misread as a zero and has resulted in serious, tenfold overdoses. Clarify any order that contains this abbreviation. Do not confuse Lantus insulin with Lente insulin.

Evaluation: Client's blood glucose levels will remain within normal range.

Drugs: Insulin Glargine (Lantus)

LANTUS

HIGH ALERT

L evel relatively constant

A lert for name confusion with lente

N ever mix with anything

T ake once a day

U ndesirable effects

S tore in cool place

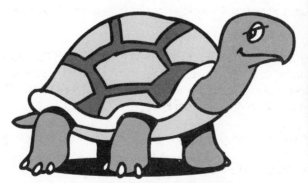

©2005 I CAN Publishing, Inc.

Lazy Lantus is in no hurry to peak. In fact, he is constant for one day or 24 hours.

MIXING INSULIN

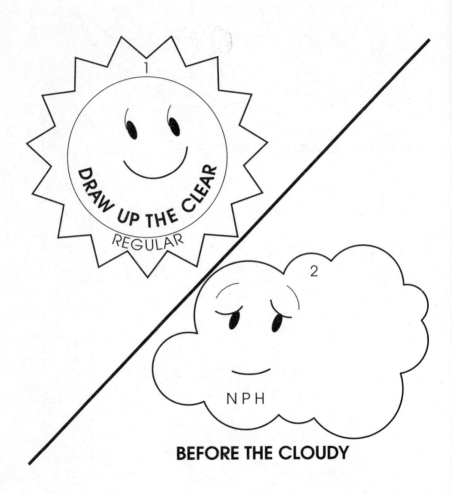

BEFORE THE CLOUDY

To prevent contaminating a short-acting insulin "**R**egular" with an intermediate insulin"**N**PH", draw the clear before the cloudy. Another way to remember is to think **RN** (**R**egistered **N**urse).

THE CONTESTANTS

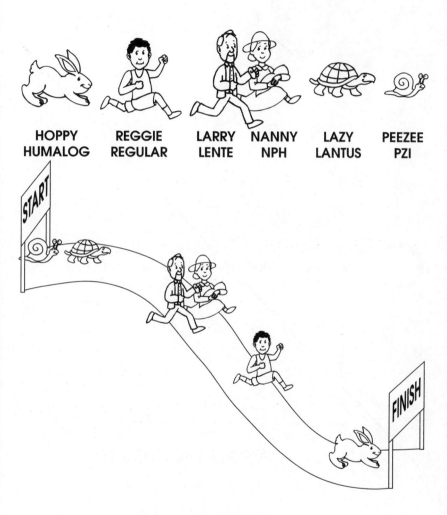

©2005 I CAN Publishing, Inc.

Insulins vary in their onset, peak and duration.

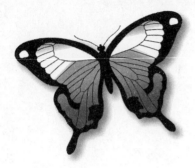

Character is like a tree and reputation its shadow. The shadow is what we think of it, the tree is the real thing.

Abraham Lincoln

Central Nervous System Agents

NONBARBITURATES SEDATIVE-HYPNOTICS

Action: CNS depression. Induces quiet, deep sleep.

Indications: Short-term treatment of insomnia.

Warnings: Hypersensitive to non-benzodiazepines. Sleep apnea. Anemia, hepatic, renal impairment, cardiac disease, gastritis, suicidal individuals, drug abuse, elderly, psychosis, seizure disorder, pregnancy, lactation, children <18 yr.

Undesirable Effects: Amnesia, daytime drowsiness, dizziness, "drugged" feeling, diarrhea, nausea, vomiting, hypersensitivity reactions, physical dependence, psychological dependence, tolerance.

Other Specific Information: Increased action of both drugs: alcohol, CNS depressants. Increased CNS depression with chamomile, kava, skullcap, valerian.

Interventions: Protect client from injury—raise bedside rails or assist with ambulation. Comply with federal narcotic laws regarding schedule IV drugs. Gastric irritations decrease by diluting dose. Baseline vital signs. Provide environment conducive to sleep. Assess sleep pattern of client. Evaluate elderly/children for paradoxical reaction. Assess blood studies, AST, ALT, bilirubin if liver damage has occurred. Assess mental status, signs of blood dyscrasias, and type of sleep problems.

Education: Take with a full glass of water or juice. Swallow whole, don't chew. Avoid alcohol and other CNS depressants. May cause dependence. Avoid abrupt discontinuation after prolonged use. Review alternative measures to improve sleep (reading, exercise several hours before hs, warm bath, warm milk, TV, self-hypnosis, etc). Clients >65 years old, usual dose 5mg.

Evaluation: Client will be able to sleep at night, decreased amount of early morning awakening if taking drug for insomnia.

Drugs: Chloral Hydrate, zolpidem (Ambien)

AMY IS NOT AN "AM BIEN"

A nxiolytic and hypnotic effects

M orning drowsiness or hangover (modulates GABA receptors to cause suppression of neurons)

B eware of drug/drug toxic effects with Rifampin (blurred vision common side effect, so avoid tasks requiring driving)

I nsomnia treatment

E ffects REM sleep pattern by suppressing it

N on-barbituate (not for long term use)

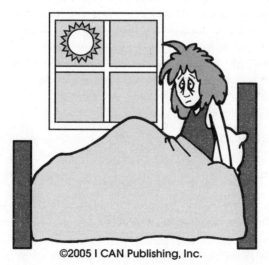

©2005 I CAN Publishing, Inc.

After Amy has taken her "AMBIEN" she goes in a deep sleep and is not ready to get up in the AM. Amy is not an "AM BIEN" (BEING).

NARCOTIC ANALGESICS

Action: Combines with opiate receptors in CNS. Reduces stimuli from sensory nerve endings; pain threshold is increased.

Indications: Moderate to severe pain, preoperative medication, and obstetrical analgesia. Methadone is used as part of heroin detoxification; hydrocodone and codeine have an antitussive effect.

Warnings: Alcoholism, respiratory, renal or hepatic disease, increased intracranial pressure, severe heart disease. Don't use Demerol in elderly patients or those with renal dysfunction.

Undesirable effects: "**Droopy Deuteronomy**" will help review the 6 D's.

Other Specific Information: Alcohol and/or CNS depressants may ↑ undesirable effects of CNS and/or respiratory depression. MAOIs may result in a fatal reaction. Note: IV doses are less than IM doses.

Interventions: Maintain records (most are class II drugs). Monitor urine output, bowel sounds, VS, and pain for type location, intensity, and duration. Dilute and administer IV solution slowly to prevent CNS depression and possible cardiac arrest. Do not mix with barbiturates. Hold medication if respirations < 12/min. with the adult or < 20/min. with the child. Have Narcan available.

Education: No alcohol or CNS depressants. Recommend nonpharmacological interventions for decreasing pain. No ambulating without assistance; no driving. Instruct to take before pain is too severe. Dependence on drug is not likely for short-term medical needs. Do not abruptly withdraw medication. Teach client with a patient-controlled analgesia (PCA) pump how to safely administer the medicine. Instruct about deep breathing and coughing, especially in clients with altered pulmonary function.

Staff Education: Do not confuse with oxycontin, oxycodone, MS Contin, morphine regular release.

Evaluation: The client's pain will be relieved without any undesirable effects from the medication.

Drugs (C-II controlled substance): Codeine; dezocine (Dalgan); fentanyl (Sublimaze); hydrocodone (Hycodan); hydromorphone (Dilaudid); levomethadyl (ORLAAM); levorphanol (Levo-Dromoran); meperidine (Demerol); methadone (Dolophine); morphine (Roxanol, MS Contin); oxycodone (Roxicodone); oxymorphone (Numorphan); propoxyphene (Darvon); remifentanil (Ultiva); sufentanil (Sufenta)

DROOPY DEUTERONOMY

HIGH ALERT

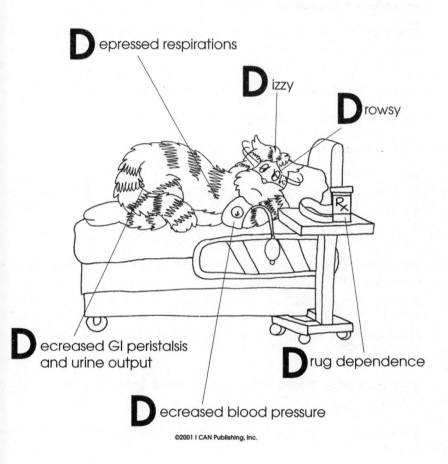

Depressed respirations

Dizzy

Drowsy

Decreased GI peristalsis and urine output

Drug dependence

Decreased blood pressure

©2001 I CAN Publishing, Inc.

"Droopy Deuteronomy" is drooping in his hospital bed from too much morphine. These drugs can make him throw up so he needs his emesis basin.

NARCOTIC ANTAGONISTS

Action: Reverses the effects of opioid agonist (narcotic analgesic) by competing for the receptor sites.

Indications: Reverses narcotic induced respiratory depression. Naloxone – drug for reversing respiratory depression.

Warnings: Hypersensitivity. Respiratory depression, narcotic addiction, cardiac disease, acute hepatitis or liver failure.

Undesirable effects: Negligible effects with no narcotics in body. The 5 P's demonstrated by "**PERKY PERKOLATOR**" will assist you in remembering these effects when the med is in the body. Pulse, pressure (blood), perspiration, pain, and puke (nausea and vomiting) are increased.

Other Specific Information: Verapamil can precipitate withdrawal in a client addicted to narcotic analgesics.

Interventions: Monitor client carefully as Naloxone "wears off" and opioid is still present; client may go back into a respiratory arrest. Nalmefene is longer acting than Naloxone, but client should still be observed until there is no risk of recurrent respiratory depression. Be aware of pain intensity when narcotic action is reversed. Have antagonist agent available. Have resuscitative equipment available immediately.

Education: Review the action of the drug with the client and family.

Evaluation: Client's respiratory rate and vital signs will remain within normal range.

Drugs: nalmefene (Revex); naloxone (Narcan); naltrexone (ReVia)

PERKY PERKOLATOR

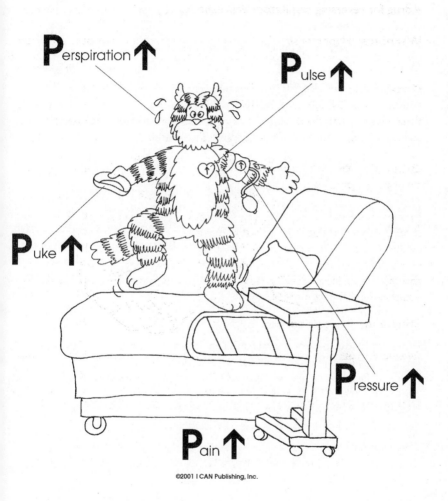

Perspiration ↑

Pulse ↑

Puke ↑

Pressure ↑

Pain ↑

©2001 I CAN Publishing, Inc.

"Perky Perkolator" is experiencing some of the undesirable effects from these drugs (the 5 P's).

CENTRAL NERVOUS SYSTEM STIMULANT
Ritalin

Action: Increases release of norepinephrine, dopamine in cerebral cortex to reticular activiting system.

Indications: Attention deficit hyperactivity disorder, narcolepsy.

Warnings: Hypersensitivity to any component in the drug; history of Tourette's disorder; history of agitation, anxious, glaucoma; caution if client has a history of depression, hypertension, drug dependency.

Undesirable Effects: Nervousness, headache, hypertension, tachycardia, insomnia, dizzy, anorexia, dry mouth, bruising (rare).

Other Specific Information: CNS stimulants may have addictive effect. MAO inhibitors may increase effect. Decreased effect of guanethidine. Increased effects of tricyclics, anticonvulsants, SSRIs. Increased stimulation with caffeine. Increased stimulation with ephedra, cola nut, guarana.

Interventions: Do not crush or allow client to chew sustained release dosage form. Administer at least 6 hr before hs to avoid sleeplessness (regular release); at least 10 hr (SR, ER). Discontinue drugs or decrease dose if paradoxical return of attention deficit disorder. Monitor B/P. Monitor CBC, urinalysis, in diabetes: blood sugar, urine sugar; insulin changes may need to be made due to a decrease in eating. Monitor height, growth rate q 3 months. Monitor mental status. Monitor for undesirable effects.

Education: Review how to take med and the appropriate time of the day. Decrease caffeine consumption. Avoid OTC preparations unless approved by provider. Taper off slowly or depression, lethargy, and increased sleeping may occur. Avoid driving if experiencing blurred vision. Avoid alcohol. Get needed rest; client will be more tired at the end of the day. Review and report undesirable effects. Dry mouth—sugarless gum, sips of tepid water.

Staff Education: Do not confuse methylphenidate with methadone. Follow standards of care when administering a Controlled Substance Schedule II medication.

Evaluation: Client will have a decrease in hyperactivity (ADD or ADHD) or ability to stay awake (narcolepsy).

Drugs: methylphenidate (Ritalin, Ritalin SR, Concerta, Metadate CD, Metadate ER, Methylin, Methylin SR, PMS-methylphenidate, Methidate, PMS-Methylphenidate, Riphenidate)

RITALIN

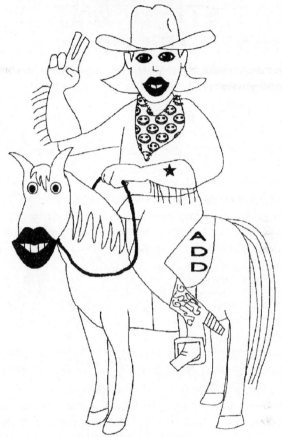

©2004 I CAN Publishing, Inc.

Avoid caffeine

Do not break, crush or chew time-released

Dopamine in cerebral cortex is increased

TexRita is on her horse ADD. Ritalin is given for attention deficit disorder.

NEUROMUSCULAR BLOCKERS

Action: Inhibits transmission of nerve impulses by binding with cholinergic receptor sites, antagonizing the action of acetylcholine.

Indications: Facilitates endotracheal intubation, skeletal muscle relaxation during mechanical ventilation, surgery, or general anesthesia.

Warnings: **HIGH ALERT DRUG** Hypersensitivity to bromide ion (Pavulon). Cardiac disease, children < 2, electrolyte imbalances, dehydration, neuromuscular disease, respiratory disease. History of malignant hyperthermia.

Undesirable Effects: Bradycardia; tachycardia; increased or decreased blood pressure; ventricular extrasystoles. Prolonged apnea, bronchospasms, cyanosis, respiratory depression. Weakness to prolonged skeletal muscle relaxation. Rash, pruritus. Anaphylaxis.

Other Specific Information: Increased neuromuscular blockade with aminoglycosides, clindamycin, enflurane, isoflurane, lincomycin, lithium, local anesthetics, opioid analgesics, polymyxin anti-infectives, quinidine, thiazides. If taken with theophylline the client may experience dysrhythmias.

Interventions: Concurrent sedation is required because of anxiety related to immobility; the client can feel, but not respond to pain. Total physical care, including ventilatory support. Cardiac monitoring including HR, BP, and ECG. Eye lubrication to prevent corneal abrasions. Interact appropriately with client and close to client since hearing is not impaired. During recovery, respirations must be assessed carefully. Neostigmine (Prostigmin) is antidote for nondepolarizing agents. Need DVT prophylaxis. Train of Four monitoring for ICU continuous infusion paralysis.

Education: Reassure client and / or family that the paralysis is only temporary. Repeat explanations about procedures and equipment due to high anxiety level.

Evaluation: The client will be paralyzed.

Drugs: atracurium (Tracrium), doxacurium (Nuromax), pancuronium (Pavulon), pipecuronium (Arduan), vecuronium (Norcuron)

RAGGEDY ANNE

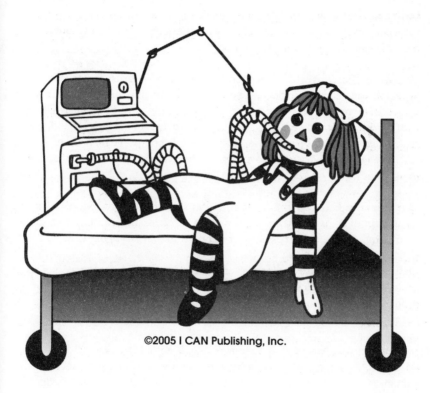

©2005 I CAN Publishing, Inc.

Raggedy Anne needs a cure. She is not unconscious but her arms and legs are falling off the table due to skeletal muscle relaxation. She can't breathe without the help of her ventilator. She has received a neuromuscular blocking agent. Many of these drugs have "curonium" in them.

ANESTHETICS— LOCAL

Action: (General) Act on the CNS to produce tranquilization and sleep before invasive procedures. Anesthetics (local) inhibit conduction of nerve impulses from sensory nerves.

Indications: General anesthetics are used to premedicate for surgery, induction and maintenance in general anesthesia. For local anesthetics, refer to individual product listing for indications.

Warnings: Persons with CVA, increased intracranial pressure, severe hypertension, cardiac decompensation should not use these products, since severe adverse reactions can occur. Use in caution with the elderly, clients with cardiovascular disease (hypotension, bradydysrhythmias), renal disease, liver disease, Parkinson's disease, children <2 yr, and pregnant women. Clients allergic to lidocaine, novocaine or bupivacaine, use chloroprocaine (Nesacaine).

Undesirable Effects: The most common side effects are dystonia, akathisia, flexion of arms, fine tremors, drowsiness, restlessness, and hypotension. Also common are chills, respiratory depression, and laryngospasm.

Other Specific Information: Metabolized in the liver and excreted in the urine. MAOIs, tricyclics, phenothiazines may cause severe hypotension or hypertension when used with local anesthetics. CNS depressants will potentiate general and local anesthetics.

Interventions: Assess VS q 10 min during IV administration, q 30 min. after IM dose. Administer anticholinergic peroperatively to decrease secretions. Administer only with crash cart, resuscitative equipment nearby. Provide a quiet environment for recovery to decrease psychotic symptoms.

Evaluation: Maintenance of anesthesia, decreased pain.

Drugs: (Injectionables only): *Local anesthetics:* lidocaine (Xylocaine), procaine (Novocaine), tetracaine (Pontocaine)

FEELINGLESS FIFI

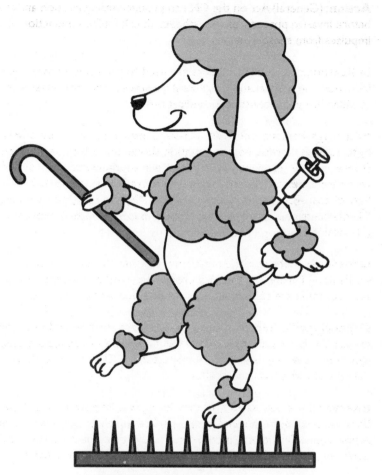

©2005 I CAN Publishing, Inc.

Fifi is walking across a bed of nails carrying her "caine" and feeling nothing. She has had an injection of a local anesthetic. Many of these anesthetics have the word **caine** in them.

MIOTICS

Action: Stimulates pupillary and ciliary sphinceter muscles resulting in pupillary constriction.

Indications: Decrease IOP in glaucoma; surgical procedures on the eye.

Warnings: Retinal detachment, ocular inflammation; avoid systemic absorption of drug with coronary artery disease, GI/GU obstruction, asthma, epilepsy.

Undesirable effects: Blurred vision, myopia, eye pain; headache; nausea, vomiting; muscle tremors; hypertension, tachycardia; retinal detachment; long term: bronchospasm.

Other Specific Information: Avoid using carbachol with pilocarpine. ↓ antiglaucoma effects with belladonna alkaloids.

Intervention: Baseline vital signs. Monitor for postural hypotension. Assess breath sounds; may develop rales or rhonchi from bronchospasm and increase bronchial secretions. Press inner canthus for a minute or two to minimize systemic absorption.

Education: Instruct client not to rinse the dropper; do not place dropper on any surface. Do not use discolored solution. Advise client not to take any atropine-like medications due to the potential increase in IOP. Instruct client and family how to safely administer eye drops. Have a return demonstration. Remember the importance of WASHING HANDS. Instruct client that long-term therapy is a possibility.

Evaluation: Intraocular pressure will return to therapeutic range.

Drugs: carbachol (Carboptic); pilocarpine (Isopto Carpine); pilocarpine nitrate (Ocusert Pilo-20, Pilo-40)

MIOTICS:
CONSTRICT EYES

MIOTICS
O
NO ATROPINE!!
S
T
R
I
C
T

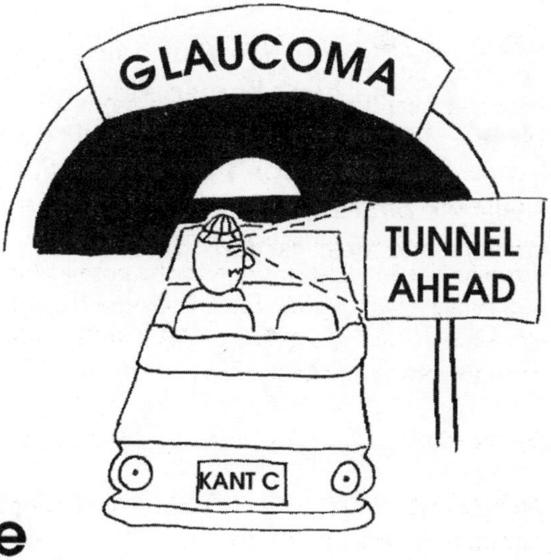

GLAUCOMA

TUNNEL
AHEAD

KANT C

CARpine
CARbachol
pilo**CAR**

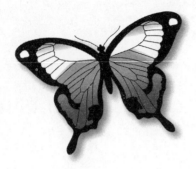

Don't go outside your house to see the flowers, my friend, don't bother with the excursion. Inside your body there are flowers. One flower has a thousand petals. That will do for a place to sit. Sitting there you will have a glimpse of beauty inside the body and out of it, before the gardens and after gardens.

Kabir

Anticonvulsant Agents

ANTICONVULSANT: DILANTIN

Action: Reduces motor cortex activity by altering transport of ions.

Indications: Grand mal and complex partial seizures.

Warnings: Hypersensitivity, heart block, psychiatric disorders.

Undesirable Effects: Nausea, vomiting, headache, diplopia, confusion, drowsiness, dizziness, ataxia, gingival hyperplasia, gingivitis, hepatitis, agranuloctyosis, red/brown discoloration of urine, male sexual dysfunction.

Other Specific Information: ↑ effects with cimetidine, chloramphenicol, isoniazid. ↓ effects of anticoagulants, antihistamines, corticosteroids, cyclosporin, dopamine, oral contraceptives, theophylline, quinidine, rifampin. *(There are numerous interactions; it is beyond the scope of this book to review all of them. We refer you to a Drug Handbook.)*

Interventions: Monitor serum drug levels (therapeutic range: 10–20 mcg/ml); labs related to renal and liver function. Provide safety during and after a seizure. If given in a suspension, shake well before pouring. If given intravenous (IV), it should be administered slowly due to potential hypotension and dysrhythmias. Administer only through a saline line. Do not mix with other drugs. Validate a good blood return.

Education: Instruct client regarding safety precautions while taking med. Inform provider of any undesirable effects. Women taking oral contraceptives may need to use an additional method of contraception. Advise female clients considering getting pregnant to consult with provider of health care since drug may have a teratogenic effect on the fetus. Do not abruptly stop the drug. Recommend preventative dental check-ups; use a soft toothbrush. Advise client that the urine may be red/brown. Discuss the importance of wearing an alert ID card and/or medic alert bracelet.

Evaluation: Client will experience less or no seizures. The serum drug level will remain therapeutic with no undesirable effects.

Drug: phenytoin (Dilantin)

DILANTIN
(DIAL AT TEN)

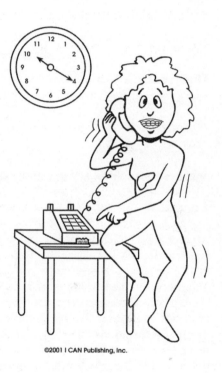

G ingival hyperplasia

U se alternate birth control

M outh care—
preventative
dental check-up

S oft tooth brush,
don't stop abruptly

©2001 I CAN Publishing, Inc.

The time is 10:20 on the clock to help you remember the therapeutic range for dilantin (10–20 mcg/ml).

ANTIEPILEPTIC AGENT: NEURONTIN

Action: Not fully understood; anticonvulsant action activity may be a result of its ability to prevent the polysynaptic responses and inhibit post-tetanic potentiation.

Indications: Combination therapy in managing partial seizures; amyotrophic lateral sclerosis. Unlabeled use: neuropathic pain.

Warnings: Hypersensitivity; lactation.

Undesirable Effects: Dizzy, insomnia, somnolence, ataxia, nervousness; nausea/vomiting; rhinitis; pruritis.

Other Specific Information: Neurontin levels will be decreased when taken with antacids.

Intervention: Arrange for support groups for epileptics.

Education: Instruct to take drug exactly as prescribed; do not abruptly make any changes without consulting provider. For nausea, recommend taking with food or milk; eat small frequent meals. Review the importance of wearing a medical alert tag identifying the medication and the fact client has epilepsy.

Evaluation: Client will experience no seizures and no undesirable effects from the drug.

Drug: gabapentin (Neurontin)

CAESAR

C NS: dizziness, insomnia—U E

A ntacids decrease

E at food with drug

S upport group for epileptics

A lert tag indicating specific drug

R eport U E

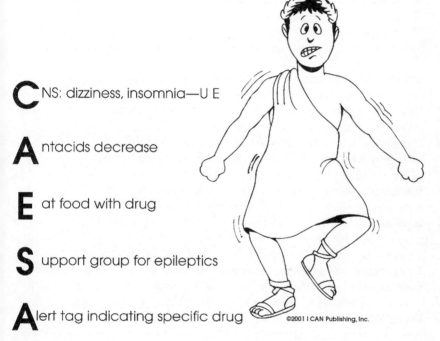

©2001 I CAN Publishing, Inc.

ANTICONVULSANT:
Valproic Acid

Action: Increases levels of GABA in the brain which decreases seizure activity.

Indications: Seizures, manic episodes associated with bipolar disorder (delayed-release only); migraine headache prevention (delayed and extended release).

Warnings: Hypersensitivity, hepatic impairment, urea cycle disorders.

Undesirable Effects: Confusion, sedation, tremor, hepatotoxicity, nausea, vomiting, abdominal cramps, diarrhea, weight gain, rash, prolonged bleeding time.

Other Specific Information: Increased risk of bleeding with antiplatelet agents, including aspirin, NSAIDs, tirofiban, eptifibatide, and abciximab, cefamandole, cefoperazone, cefotetan, heparins, and thrombolytic agents or warfarin. Additive CNS depression with CNS depressants, alcohol, antihistamines, antidepressants, opioid analgesics, MAO inhibitors, and sedative / hypnotics.

Interventions: Monitor hepatic function (LDH, AST, ALT, and bilirubin) and serum ammonia concentrations, especially during initial 6 months of therapy; fatalities from liver failure have occurred. Discontinue if hyperammonemia occurs. Therapeutic levels range from 50–100 micrograms per ml. Monitor mental status, respiratory status. Tablets or capsules whole; do not crush, break, or chew. Elixir alone; do not dilute with carbonated beverage; do not give syrup to client on a sodium restriction. Give with food or milk.

Education: Review that physical dependency may result from extended use. Avoid driving and other activities that require alertness. Do not discontinue after long-term use; convulsions my result. Report undesirable effects to provider of care.

Evaluation: Client will experience decreased seizure activity or decreased manic behavior, or frequency of migraine headaches.

Drugs: valproic acid (Depakote, Depakote ER, Depakene, Epival)

VALPROIC ACID

D iscontinue if hyperammonemia occurs

E levate levels of GABA in brain

P rolonged bleeding if given with antiplatelet agents

A void CNS depressants and don't give
wth carbonated beverages

C
O
Y
O
T
E

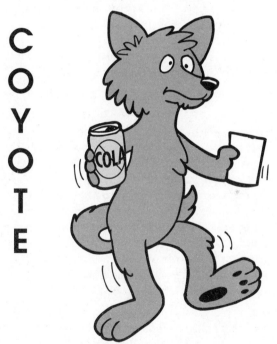

©2005 I CAN Publishing, Inc.

Coty Coyote may be shaking from mania, seizures or his head may be pounding from a migraine. Depakote treats these symptoms but should not be given with carbonated beverages. Milk helps prevent GI upset.

ANTICONVULSANT:
Carbamazepine

Action: Inhibits nerve impulses by limiting influx of sodium ions into the motor cortex from across the cell membrane.

Indications: Tonic-clonic, complex-partial, mixed seiqures; trigeminal neuralgia, diabetic neuropathy. Mood stabilizers. Alternative to lithium or valproic acid or adjunctive treatment for bipolar disorder.

Warnings: Hypersensitivity to this category or tricyclics, bone marrow depression, MAOIs. Glaucoma, hepatic, renal or cardiac disease.

Other Specific Information: CNS toxicity when taken with lithium. Increased carbamazepine levels with cimetidine, clarithromycin, danazol, diltiazem, erythromycin, fluoxetine, fluvoxamine, isoniazid, propoxyphene, valproic acid, verapamil. Decreased effects of benzodiazepines, doxycycline, felbate, haloperidol, oral contracteptives, phenobarbital, phenytoin, primidone, theophylline, thyroid hormones, warfarin. Increased levels of desmopressin, lithium, lypressin, vasopressin. Fatal reaction with MAOIs. Increased peak concentration of carbamazepine with grapefruit juice.

Undesirable Effects: Anorexia, nausea, dizziness, sedation, headache, dry mouth, constipation, rash.

Interventions: For seizures, identify and document the character, duration, location, frequency, and presence of an aura. For trigeminal neuralgia document the characteristics of the facial pain. Monitor renal studies, ALT, AST, bilirubin. Blood studies (hgb, hct, RBC) should be evaluated q month. Maintain drug level between 4–12 micrograms/ml. Anorexia may indicate increased blood levels. Notify provider if mood, sensorium, affect or any behavioral changes occur. Monitor eyes by ophthalmic examinations before, during, and after treatment. Discontinue if client experiences purpura or a red raised rash. Blood dyscrasias may present with a sore throat, fever, bruising, rash, and/or jaundice. Report immediately. May take med with food, milk to reduce GI distress. Do not crush, break, or chew ext. rel. tab; chewable tabs: tell client to chew tab, not swallow it whole; ext. rel. cap may be opened and mixed with food.

Education: Carry emergency ID identifying client's name, drugs currently taken, condition, health care provider's name, phone number. Avoid driving or any activities that require alertness for a minimum of 3 days to determine the response from the medication. Do not quickly discontinue the medication after long-term use. Report any undesirable effects.

Evaluation: Client will experience decreased seizure activity.

Drug: carbamazepine (Apo-Carbamazepine, Atretol, Carbatrol, Epitol, Novo-Carbamaz, Tegretol, Tegretol CR, Tegretol-XR)

CARBAMAZEPINE

T rigeminial Neuralgia, Tonic-clonic seizures

E valuate for UE; anorexia, nausea, dizziness, sedation, headache, sore throat

G ive with food, milk to reduce GI distress

R eview levels, maintain—between 4-12 micrograms/ml

E valuate for anorexia—may indicate toxic levels

T ablet—chewable; do not swallow whole, chew. Take extended-release capsules whole—no crushing or breaking

O pen & mix with food—extended-release capsules

L ook for MANY drug/drug interactions

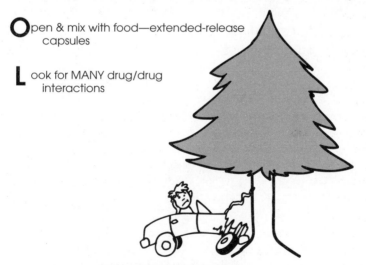

©2005 I CAN Publishing, Inc.

Remember the CAR BAMA (banged at) ZE (the) PINE tree. An undesirable effect of this drug could be sedation and dizziness. Before operating any dangerous equipment or driving an automobile, clients need to determine their response to the drug.

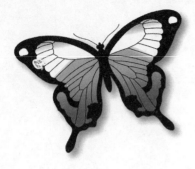

Our lives improve only when we take chances—and the first and most difficult risk we can take is to be honest with ourselves.

Walter Anderson

Anxiolytics, Antidepressants, and Antipsychotic Agents

ANTIANXIETY:
BENZODIAZEPINES

Action: Appears to enhance action of gamma-aminobutyric acid (GABA inhibitory neurotransmitter). Depresses the limbic and subcortical CNS.

Indications: Anxiety, preoperative medication, and skeletal muscle relaxant. Versed is commonly used for induction of anesthesia and sedation prior to diagnostic tests and endoscopic exams. Klonopin is used primarily as an anticonvulsant. Ativan and Librium for alcohol withdrawal.

Warnings: Hypersensitivity, renal or hepatic dysfunction, mental depression, pregnancy, lactation, glaucoma, young children, addiction-prone, 14 days within a MAO inhibitor. Caution in the elderly, debilitated, or client with COPD. Ativan clearance less affected by hepatic dysfunction than other benzodiazepines.

Undesirable Effects: The 3 D's that most frequently occur are **d**rowsiness, **d**izziness, and **d**ecreased blood pressure. When taken alone, there is a low incidence of toxicity. Rare effects include: **d**ependence on drug, **d**epressed respirations, liver **d**ysfunction and blood **d**yscrasias (4 D's).

Other Specific Information: CNS depressants, especially alcohol, may result in ↑ sedation. ↑ effect with cimetidine, disulfiram, omeprazole, oral contraceptives.

Interventions: Monitor VS, cardiovascular status, mental status; liver function tests and blood counts with clients on long-term therapy. Assess for symptoms of leukopenia (i.e. fever, sore throat). Provide a restful environment if giving IV infusion. Consider for abuse and dependence. If given IV, have respiratory equipment available; keep client recumbent. Do not mix antianxiety drugs with other drugs in a syringe. Safety precautions for drowsiness. Flumazenil (Rocmazicon) is approved for benzodiazepine overdose.

Education: Recommend small frequent meals. Encourage to rise slowly from supine position and dangle feet prior to standing. Avoid alcohol, smoking and other CNS depressants. Avoid activities needing good psychomotor coordination until CNS effects are known. May cause physical or psychological dependence. Avoid abrupt discontinuation after prolonged use. Providers, including dentists should be advised that client is taking this medication. Review methods to control excess stress and anxiety. Advise client to wear medical alert indicating drug therapy.

Evaluation: Client will be less anxious and will be able to cope with the daily stressors in life.

Drugs: (C-IV controlled substance) alprazolam (Xanax); chlordiazepoxide (Librium); clonazepam (Klonopin); clorazepate (Tranxene); diazepam (Valium); lorazepam (Ativan); midazolam (Versed); oxazepam (Serax)

ANTIANXIETY

A void abrupt discontinuation after prolonged use

N ot give if ↑ BP, renal/hepatic dysfunction or hx of drug abuse

X anax, Ativan, Serax—a few examples

I ncrease in 3D's—drowsiness, dizziness, decreased BP

E nhances action of GABA (inhibitory transmitter)

T each to rise slowly from supine

Y es, alcohol should be avoided

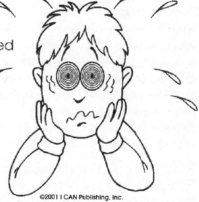

©2001 I CAN Publishing, Inc.

MISCELLANEOUS ANTIANXIETY AGENTS: NONBENZODIAZEPINES

Action: Interacts with serotonin and dopamine at presynaptic neurotransmitter receptors in the CNS, resulting in an antianxiety effect.

Indications: Short term relief management (up to 4 wks.) of anxiety and anxiety disorders. Nonaddicting: used to avoid benzodiazepines and barbiturates.

Warnings: Hypersensitivity to buspirone or any components. Renal/ hepatic impairment, MAO inhibitor therapy; pregnancy/lactation.

Undesirable Effects: Dizziness, drowsiness, headache, nausea, fatigue. Insomnia, blurred vision, and confusion are experienced less frequently.

Other Specific Information: Alcohol or CNS depressants may ↑ sedation. MAO inhibitors may ↑ blood pressure. ↓ effects with fluoxetine when given with Buspar. Refer to tricyclic antidepressants for drug interactions with Sinequan.

Interventions: Monitor level of anxiety, mental status, neuromuscular coordination, and vital signs. Offer support for anxious client. Assist with ambulating if drowsy or dizzy.

Education: Inform client that it may take 1–2 weeks of therapy before the effects are present. Therapeutic effect generally takes 3–4 weeks of therapy. Avoid any task requiring alertness until established response of drug. Avoid alcohol and other CNS depressants (unless ordered by provider). Recommend taking medication with food. Do not abruptly discontinue this drug.

Evaluation: Client's behavior will reflect less anxiety with no undesirable effects from the medication.

Drugs: buspirone (Buspar); doxepin (Sinequan); meprobamate (Miltown, Equanil)

BUSPAR BUS

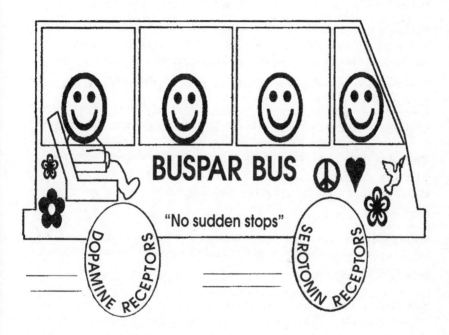

Get on the Buspar Bus to decrease ansiety. The seats recline for the undesirable effect of dizziness and drowsiness. Smiles can be seen after taking the drug for a week.

CONCEPT: DEPRESSION

Driving is out until response to drug has been determined: Since some of the undesirable effects from these medications include sedation, drowsiness, hypotension, and blurred vision, instruct client not to drive. Recommend that client determines the response of the drug dose prior to operating hazardous machinery.

Effect has a delayed onset of 7–21 days: Client needs to be informed that the effectiveness of these drugs may take 7–21 days. Client may get frustrated prior to this, so it is important to share this information.

Planning pregnancy—consult with provider of care: Due to the potential teratogenic effects of the drug on the fetus, it is recommended that the client not get pregnant while taking these medications.

Relieves symptoms, not a CURE: Recommend counseling to assist with the depression.

Evaluate vital signs: Orthostatic hypotension is common. Anticholinergic like symptoms may occur such as dry mouth, urinary retention, blurred vision, increased heart rate, and constipation. Evaluate weight several times a week.

Stopping drug abruptly is OUT: Client needs to understand the importance of this.

Safety measures (i.e., change position slowly): Instruct the client to come to a standing position slowly to avoid feeling faint from orthostatic hypotension.

Instruct client to report undesirable effects: Inform client to report anticholinergic effects of the drugs, such as dry mouth and eyes, blurred vision, constipation, and urinary retention. Since dry mouth is a common undesirable effect, encourage client to practice good oral hygiene to prevent dental caries. Ice chips, breath mints, and sugarless candies are also effective in promoting comfort.

Observe for suicidal tendencies: The risk of suicide is typically higher near the end of the depression cycle. Client needs to be monitored for suicidal tendencies.

No alcohol or CNS depressants: Instruct client to avoid alcoholic beverages or other CNS depressants while taking antidepressants because CNS depression may be increased.

Anxiolytics, Antidepressants, and Antipsychotic Agents

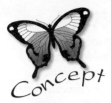

Concept

ANTIDEPRESSANTS

D riving is out until response to drug has been determined

E ffect has a delayed onset of 7–21 days

P lanning pregnancy—consult with provider of care

R elieves symptoms, not a CURE!

E valuate vital signs

S topping drug abruptly is OUT!

S afety measures (i.e., change position slowly)

I nstruct client to report undesirable effects

O bserve for suicidal tendencies

N o alcohol or CNS depressants

©2001 I CAN Publishing, Inc.

SELECTIVE SEROTONIN REUPTAKE INHIBITORS (SSRIs)

Action: Causes selective inhibition of serotonin uptake resulting in an antidepressant response.

Indications: Depression, obsessive-compulsive disorder, panic disorder, and appetite disorders.

Warnings: Renal or hepatic function impairments. Seizures, mania, cardiac disease, pregnancy/lactation, or within 14 days of MAOIs.

Undesirable Effects: "**CNS**" will help you recall these effects. **C**NS stimulation-headache, insomnia, nervousness, agitation. **N**ausea, anorexia, diarrhea, vomiting. **S**kin rash, sexual dysfunction. (SSRIs are **less** likely than the other antidepressants to cause anticholinergic effects, cardiotoxicity, sedation, seizures, as well as inducing mania in bipolar clients.)

Other Specific Information: Avoid use with highly protein-bound drugs (e.g., warfarin), within 14 days of MAOIs, alcohol, caution with CNS depressants. Antacids may ↓ absorption. Use cautiously with type IC antiarrhythmics due to potential drug interactions. ↑ risk of reaction if combined with St. John's Wort.

Interventions: For long-term therapy, liver/renal function tests should be monitored. Blood tests should be performed periodically. Monitor PT and INR with clients receiving concurrent warfarin therapy. Monitor BP, HR, weight, and stools for consistency. A rash, especially with a temperature, should be reported immediately. Monitor elderly for fluid and sodium imbalance. If client experiences dizziness, assist with ambulation.

Education: Advise client to take medication in the morning to avoid insomnia. To obtain maximum therapeutic response, it may require 3- 4 weeks of therapy (in the elderly, it may take 10-12 weeks of therapy). Advise clients on warfarin therapy to promptly report signs of bleeding. (Refer to "**DEPRESSION**".)

Evaluation: Client has improvement in clinical state (i.e., appearance, behavior, interest, mood, speech patterns).

Drugs: citalopram (Celexa); fluoxetine (Prozac); fluvoxamine (Luvox); paroxetine (Paxil); sertraline (Zoloft), escitalopram (Lexapro)

Anxiolytics, Antidepressants, and Antipsychotic Agents

PAXIL

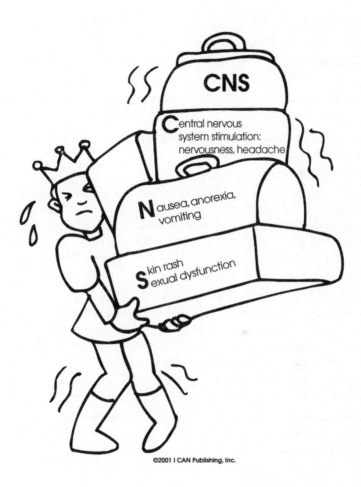

CNS

Central nervous system stimulation: nervousness, headache

Nausea, anorexia, vomiting

Skin rash **S**exual dysfunction

©2001 I CAN Publishing, Inc.

Paxil packs extra baggage when taking SSRIs. The baggage will help you remember some of the major undesirable effects from these medications.

TRICYCLIC ANTIDEPRESSANTS

Action: Blocks re-uptake of norepinephrine and serotonin into nerve endings.

Indications: Depression. Imipramine is also used for childhood enuresis. Clomipramine is used for obsessive-compulsive disorders.

Warnings: Epilepsy, glaucoma, cardiovascular disease, urinary retention, seizures, hyperthyroidism, pregnancy/lactation, within 14 days of receiving MAOIs.

Undesirable Effects: Manic signs in bipolar clients. Refer to "**HATS**" to help remember these effects. **H**ypotension, **A**nticholinergic effects, **T**achycardia, and **S**edation.

Other Specific Information: Oral contraceptives may alter tricyclic serum levels. ↑ effect of alcohol, CNS depressants, adrenergic agents, and anticholinergics. Antithyroid agents may ↑ risk of agranulocytosis. Phenothiazines may ↑ sedative effects. Cimetidine may ↑ toxicity. If taking sympathomimetics, may ↑ cardiac effect. If taking MAO inhibitors, may ↑ risk of hypertensive crisis, convulsion. Do not give TCAs with MAOIs.

Interventions: Monitor periodic blood cell counts, glaucoma tests, hepatic and renal function studies. When evaluating the drug level, blood samples should be taken immediately before the first morning dose or at least 8 hours after a dose. Monitor BP and HR at appropriate intervals. Manic or hypomanic episodes may occur with cyclic types of disorders. May need to discontinue tricyclics until episode is relieved.

Education: Instruct client if sedation is problematic, a single dose at bedtime may be beneficial. Due to adverse interactions with anesthetic agents, instruct client to discontinue the TCAs 2–3 days prior to surgery. (Refer to "**DEPRESSION**".)

Evaluation: Client has improvement in clinical state (i.e. appearance, behavior, effects, interest, mood, speech patterns).

Drugs: amitriptyline (Elavil); amoxapine (Asendin); clomipramine (Anafranil); desipramine (Norpramin); doxepin (Adapin, Sinequan); imipramine (Tofranil); nortriptyline (Aventyl, Pamelor); protriptyline (Vivactil); trimipramine (Surmontil)

TINA TRICYCLE

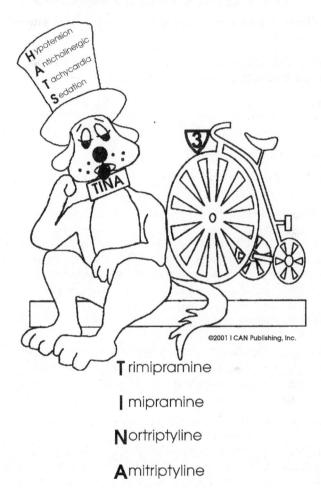

Hypotension
Anticholinergic
Tachycardia
Sedation

TINA

©2001 I CAN Publishing, Inc.

T rimipramine

I mipramine

N ortriptyline

A mitriptyline

Tina Tricycle is sitting on the curb as she is sleepy and can't pee, can't see, can't spit nor can't shit. Obviously she should not be driving "heavy machinery" while taking tricyclic antidepressants. The 3 wheels of the ticycle will help you remember that the therapeutic effects may have a 3 week delay of onset. After her body adjusts to the meds she may be able to ride again. "HATS" are some of the other undesirable effects she may experience.

MONOAMINE OXIDASE INHIBITOR (MAOI)

Action: Inhibits the enzyme (MAO) that breaks down norepinephrine and serotonin.

Indications: Second or third line drugs for the depression. These are effective, but are more dangerous than others.

Warnings: Alcoholism, congestive heart failure, pheochromocytoma, history of headache, uncontrolled hypertension, hepatic/renal impairment. Do not give Demerol.

Undesirable effects: Orthostatic hypotension. Hypertensive crisis if food containing tyramine is eaten. CNS effects: agitation, headache. Anticholinergic effects. Photosensitivity.

Other Specific Information: Hypertensive crisis within several hours of ingestion of a tyramine-containing product. Parnate is the most likely drug to cause this problem and the onset is rapid. Avoid foods containing tyramine such as aged cheese, beer, ale, red wine, pickled foods, smoked or pickled fish, beef or chopped liver, avocados, or figs. Tricyclic antidepressants, fluoxetine, and trazodone may cause serotonin syndrome.

Interventions: Monitor periodic liver function tests and ongoing VS. Assess for needed emotional support. Discontinue immediately with hypertensive crisis. Phentolamine mesylate (Regitine) should be on hand to control a severe hypertension reaction.

Education: After stopping the MAOI, instruct client to wait 2–3 weeks prior to taking another antidepressant. Review products high in tyramine. Administer in AM to avoid insomnia. Notify provider for signs of hypertensive crisis. Recommend wearing a medical identification band indicating MAOI therapy. Inform provider about the MAOI if dental or emergency care is needed. Usually discontinue MAOIs 10 days prior to surgery. (Refer to "**DEPRESSION**".)

Evaluation: Client has improvement in clinical state (i.e., appearance, behavior, interest, mood, speech patterns).

Drugs: isocarboxazid (Marplan); phenelzine (Nardil); tranylcypromine (Parnate)

Anxiolytics, Antidepressants, and Antipsychotic Agents

THE "TYRANT" KING

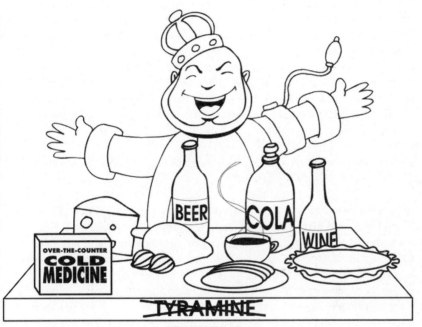

©2001 I CAN Publishing, Inc.

The "tyrant" king loves good food, but can develop a life threatening hypertensive crisis if he eats or drinks products containing **TYRAMINE** while taking MAO inhibitors. The "tyrant" is **N**o **P**opular **M**an (**N**ardil, **P**arnate, **M**arplan [*this will help you remember MAO inhibitors*]).

OTHER ANTIDEPRESSANTS

Action: Inhibits reuptake of dopamine, serotonin, norepinephrine.

Indications: Depression, Wellbutin also is used for smoking cessation.

Warnings: Convulsive disorders, prostatic hypertrophy, severe renal, hepatic, cardiac disease depending on the type of medication. Use cautiously in suicidal clients, severe depression, schizophrenia, hyperactivity, diabetes mellitus, and the elderly.

Undesirable Effects: Dizziness, drowsiness, diarrhea, dry mouth, decrease urinary output (from retention), and decrease in the blood pressure from orthostatic hypotension. "GOATS" on the next page will assist you in remembering the major undesirable effects. They are minimal, however, in comparison to the other categories of antidepressants. GI effects are actually the major effects with these drugs.

Other Specific Information: Refer to individual monographs since interactions vary widely among products.

Interventions: Monitor B/P (lying, standing), pulse q 4 h; if systolic B/P drops 20 mm HG, hold drug, notify provider. Monitor blood studies, AST, ALT, bilirubin, creatinine, weight. Monitor for EPS in elderly clients. Monitor mental status, urinary retention, constipation. Do not discontinue abruptly. If alcohol is consumed hold drug until AM. Increase fluids for urinary retention and bulk in diet if constipation occurs. If GI symptoms occur, administer with food or milk. Gum, hard candy or frequent sips of water for dry mouth. Assistance with ambulation while beginning therapy. Safety measures including side rails primarily in elderly. Check to see if PO medication is swallowed.

Education: Teach that therapeutic effects may take 2–3 weeks. Use caution with driving due to drowsiness, dizziness or blurred vision. Avoid alcohol or other CNS depressants. Do not discontinue quickly.

Evaluation: Client will have a decrease in depression.

Drugs: amoxapine (Asendin), bupropion (Wellbutrin, Wellbutrin SR), maprotiline (Ludiomil, Novartis), mirtazapine (Remeron Organon), nefazodone (Serzone), trazodone (Desyrel, Apothecon), venlafaxine (Effexor/Effexor XR)

Anxiolytics, Antidepressants, and Antipsychotic Agents

GOATS

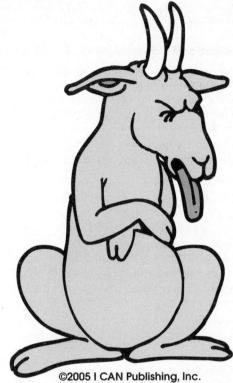

©2005 I CAN Publishing, Inc.

G I distress

O rthostatic hypotension

A nticholinergic effects (can't see, pee, spit, shit)

agi **T** ation/insomnia

S edation
sexual dysfunction

The goat is sitting to prevent falling from low blood pressure. His expression indicates his agitation, but he doesn't have enough energy to run.

ANTIMANIC MEDICATION

Action: Inhibits release of norepinephrine and dopamine. Alters sodium transport in nerve and muscle cells.

Indications: Manic episodes of manic-depressive (Bipolar) disorder.

Warnings: Cardiovascular disease, renal disease, severe dehydration, thyroid disease, elderly.

Undesirable Effects: *Minor toxicity*: nausea, vomiting, diarrhea, GI upset, fine hand tremors, thirst, polyuria. *Mild to moderate toxicity*: coarse tremors, confusion, ataxia, blurred vision, diluted urine, severe polydipsia, tinnitus. *Life threatening*: Cardiac dysrhythmias, circulatory collapse.

Other Specific Information: ↑ risk of toxicity when given with thiazide diuretics, methyldopa, and NSAIDS. ↓ lithium levels with excess sodium and antacids. ↑ CNS toxicity with haloperidol. There is a narrow therapeutic index. (.6–1.2 mEq/L: therapeutic), (> 1.5mEq/L: toxic), (2.0mEq/L: lethal).

Interventions: Therapeutic levels for maintenance are 0.6–1.2 mEq/L. Long term levels should be maintained below 0.9 mEq/L. Evaluate levels every 3–4 days during initial phase of therapy, every 1–2 months thereafter, and weekly if no improvement of mania or undesirable effects continue to occur. Blood samples taken just before the AM dose when there is a maximum stabilization of the serum concentration. Monitor fluid status, serum electrolytes, and renal function. Pre-treatment exam—thyroid, kidney function testing and EKG. Assess serum lithium levels daily with severe renal or cardiovascular disease, dehydration, and debilitation. Supervise suicidal risk. Monitor for undesirable effects. Management of lithium toxicity: osmotic diuretic.

Education: Teach symptoms of lithium toxicity. Avoid tasks requiring psychomotor coordination until CNS effects are known. Maintain a steady salt and fluid intake (2.5 to 3 liters per day; especially in summer). Administer with meals. Avoid caffeine.

Evaluation: Client is free of manic-depressive disorder as demonstrated by an improved mental status.

Drugs: Lithium Carbonate (Eskalith, Lithobid, Lithonate)

Anxiolytics, Antidepressants, and Antipsychotic Agents

BIPOLAR CLOWN

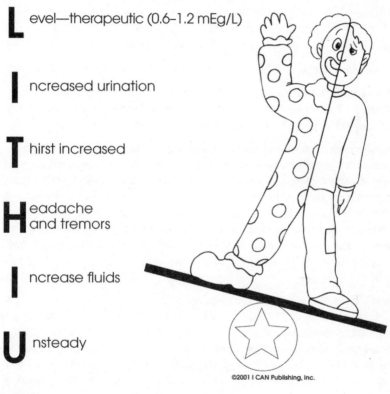

L evel—therapeutic (0.6–1.2 mEg/L)

I ncreased urination

T hirst increased

H eadache and tremors

I ncrease fluids

U nsteady

M orton's Salt—adequate intake

©2001 I CAN Publishing, Inc.

ANTIPSYCHOTICS

Action: Blocks dopamine receptor sites in the brain. There is a depression of the limbic system and cerebral cortex that controls aggression. Antiemetic effects by inhibiting the chemoreceptor trigger zones in the medulla. May initiate anticholinergic, antihistamine and/or sedative effects.

Indications: Schizophrenic disorders; mania; agitated organic disorders; delusional disorders. Antiemetic; intractable hiccups. Preoperative sedation (i.e., Compazine, Phenergan).

Warnings: Alcoholism, or other CNS depression; hepatic, renal, or coronary disease; cerebral insufficiency; severe hypotension; glaucoma; bone marrow depression; blood dyscrasias; young children. Use cautiously in elderly and debilitated clients.

Undesirable Effects: "**STANCE**" on the next page will help you remember these effects.

Other Specific Information: Alcohol, CNS depressants may ↑ CNS and respiratory de-pression. Tricyclics and MAO inhibitors may ↑ sedation, hypotensive and anticholinergic effects. ↓ levodopa effects. Lithium, antacids, and antidiarrheals may ↓ absorption.

Interventions: Monitor periodic liver function studies, WBCs, serum glucose, VS, and psy-chological assessments during therapy. Orthostatic hypotension is likely to occur; rise slowly with assistance and initiate safety measures. Suicidal precautions if necessary. Do not mix parenteral solutions with other drugs in same syringe. Give deep IM injection. Following parenteral route, remain in supine position for at least 30 minutes. Liquid should be protected from light and should be diluted with fruit juice before administering. Avoid skin contact with oral suspension solution. Treat extrapyramidal symptoms with anticholinergics (i.e., Cogentin). Discontinue at least 48 hours before surgery.

Education: Teach that urine may turn pink or reddish brown. Advise that the medication may take 6 wks or longer to achieve a full therapeutic effect. Instruct to give daily dose 1–2 hours before bedtime. Oral concentrate must be diluted in 2–3 oz. of liquid (water, fruit juice, carbonated drink, milk, or pudding). Avoid sun exposure (use sun block). Caution against driving a car or operating machinery. Explain the importance of reporting a sore throat, fever, or symptoms of infection. Undesirable effects usually subside within approximately 2 weeks of therapy or decrease by dose adjustment. Inform other providers when taking these drugs. Advise client to wear an ID bracelet indicating the medication therapy.

Evaluation: The client is able to cope with and perform activities of daily living independently.

Drugs: *Phenothiazines:* chlorpromazine (Thorazine); fluphenazine (Prolixin); mesoridazine (Serentil); perphenazine (Trilafon); prochlorperazine (Compazine); promazine (Sparine); thio-ridazine (Mellaril); trifluoperazine (Stelazine); triflupromazine (Vesprin); ***Nonphenothiazines:*** clozapine (Clozaril); haloperidol (Haldol); loxapine (Loxitane); molindone (Moban); olanzap-ine (Zyprexa); pimozide (Orap); quetiapine (Seroquel); risperidone (Risperdal); thiothixene (Navane)

Anxiolytics, Antidepressants, and Antipsychotic Agents

STANCE

S edation
sunlight sensitivity

T ardive dyskinesia
achycardia
remors

A nticholinergic
granulocytosis
ddiction

N euroleptic malignant syndrome

C ardiac arrhythmias (orthostatic hypotension)

E xtrapyramidal (akathesia)
ndocrine (change in libido)

©2001 I CAN Publishing, Inc.

STANCE will help you remember the undesirable effects of Antipsychotics.

ATYPICAL ANTIPSYCHOTIC

Action: Atypical antipsychotic/neuroleptic. Benzisoxazole derivative. Exact mechanism unknown. Dopamine and serotonin receptor antagonists.

Indications: More effective for negative symptoms of schizophrenia (amotivation, affect, isolation).

Warnings: Hypersensitivity, lactation, seizure disorders, renal disease, hepatic disease, children, pregnancy, and the elderly.

Undesirable Effects: Newest agent in class (as such, minimal published clinical trial data); transient nausea, vomiting possible; anxiety and insomnia also reported; minimal to no prolactin elevation, QT prolongation, or weight gain. While the image on the next page is the same as the image for the typical antipsychotics, the undesirable effects in "STANCE" are very low for this drug.

Other Specific Information: Increased effects of aripiprazole: CYP3A4 inhibitors (ketoconazole), CYP2D6 inhibitors (quinidine, fluoxetine, paroxetine); reduce dose of aripiprazole. Increased sedation: other CNS depressants and alcohol. Increased EPS with other antipsychotics, lithium. Decreased effects of aripiprazole: CYP3A4 inducers (carbamazepine), increased dose of aripiprazole. Increased CNS depression with kava.

Interventions: Assess mental status prior to initiating drug. I&O. Monitor bilirubin, CBC, LFTs every month. Assess affect, LOC, gait, sleep pattern, etc. Monitor blood pressure standing and lying; also heart rate, respirations. Report drops of 30 mmHg in B/P; assess for ECG changes. Monitor dizziness, faintness, tachycardia on rising. Monitor EPS, including akathesia, tardive dyskinesia (bizarre movements of the jaw, mouth, tongue, extremities), pseudoparkinsonism. Assess for neuroleptic malignant syndrome; hyperthermia, increased CPK , altered mental status, muscle rigidity. Assess skin turgor daily along with constipation, urinary retention. Supervise ambulation until client is stabilized on the med. Decrease stimulus by dimming lights and avoiding loud environmental sounds.

Education: Advise client about orthostatic hypotension and how to handle rising from sitting or lying. Recommend avoiding hot tubs, hot showers, tub baths due to hypotension. Avoid abruptly withdrawing the drug. EPS may result. Withdraw slowly. Avoid OTC preparation unless approved by provider of care. Avoid hazardous activities if drowsy or dizzy. Report impaired vision, tremors, muscle twitching. In hot weather, take precautions to remain cool.

Evaluation: Client will experience a decrease in emotional excitement, hallucinations, delusions, paranoia. There will be evidence of a reorganization of patterns of thought and speech.

Drug: aripiprazole (Ablify)

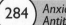

Anxiolytics, Antidepressants, and Antipsychotic Agents

STANCE

S edation
sunlight sensitivity

T ardive dyskinesia
achycardia
remors

A nticholinergic
granulocytosis
ddiction

N euroleptic malignant syndrome

C ardiac arrhythmias (orthostatic hypotension)

E xtrapyramidal (akathesia)
ndocrine (change in libido)

©2001 I CAN Publishing, Inc.

GEODON

Action: Unknown: may be mediated through both dopamine type 2 (D2) and serotonin type 2 (5-HT2) antagonism. Benzisoxazole derivative.

Indications: Antipsychotic/neuroleptic. Schizophrenia, acute agitation.

Warnings: Hypersensitivity, lactation, seizure activity.

Undesirable Effects: EPS, pseudoparkinsonism, akathesia, dystonia, tardive dyskinesia; drowsiness, insomnia, agitation, headache, seizures, neuroleptic malignant sydrome, dizzy, tremor. Orthostatic hypotension, tachycardia, sudden death. Anorexia, constipation, weight gain, dry mouth, rhinitis.

Other Specific Information: Increased sedation with other CNS depressants, alcohol. Increased EPS with other antipsychotics, lithium. Increased excretion of ziprasidone: carbamazepine. Increased ziprasidone with ketoconazole. Increased hypotension with antihypertensives. Increased CNS depression with chamomile, kava, skullcap, or valerian.

Interventions: Assess mental status prior to initiating the drug. Assess I&O; palplate bladder if urinary output is low. Every month monitor Bilirubin, CBC, LFTs. Assess affect, orientation, LOC, etc. Assess B/P standing and lying; also heart rate, respirations. Monitor for undesirable effects. Decrease stimuli by dimming lights; provide a quiet environment. Supervise ambulation until client is stabilized on the medication. Increase fluids to decrease constipation.

Education: Instruct to take capsule whole and do not open or crush. Advise to take with food. Review the importance of rising from sitting or lying position gradually due to orthostatic hypotension. Avoid hot baths. Advise not to abruptly withdraw the drug due to EPS. Withdraw drug slowly. Avoid OTC preparations of cold, cough, hay fever medicine, alcohol, and CNS depressants. Report undesirable effects. In hot weather, take precautions to remain cool.

Evaluation: Client will have a decrease in emotional excitement, hallucinations, delusions, paranoia; reorganization of thinking process and speech.

Drug: ziprasidone (Geodon)

STANCE

S edation
sunlight sensitivity

T ardive dyskinesia
tachycardia
tremors

A nticholinergic
agranulocytosis
addiction

N euroleptic malignant syndrome

C ardiac arrhythmias (orthostatic hypotension)

E xtrapyramidal (akathesia)
endocrine (change in libido)

©2001 I CAN Publishing, Inc.

Notice Stance has a doubled up fist because he is agitated. This drug may cause sensitivity to sun light. Geodon will help control this feeling.

ANTI-ALZHEIMER'S AGENT: ARICEPT

Action: Elevates acetylcholine concentrations (cerebral cortex) by slowing degradation of acetylcholine released in cholinergic neurons. Reversible cholinesterase inhibitor.

Indications: Mild to moderate dementia in Alzheimer's disease.

Warnings: Hypersensitivity to donepezil or piperidine derivatives. Sick sinus syndrome, history of ulcers, GI bleeding, hepatic disease, bladder obstruction, asthma, COPD, seizures.

Undesirable Effects: Headaches, abnormal dreams, dizziness, drowsiness, depression, fatigue, insomnia, syncope, atrial fibrillation, hypertension, hypotension, vasodilation, diarrhea, nausea, anorexia, vomiting, frequent urination, hot flashes, ecchymoses, arthritis, muscle cramps.

Other Specific Information: Exaggerates muscle relaxation from succinylcholine. Increased drug-drug interactions with anticholinergics and theophylline. When taken with NSAIDs, there is an increased gastric acid secretion. Decreased donepezil effect: carbamazepine, dexamethasone, phenytoin, phenobarbital, rifampin.

Interventions: Monitor pulse during therapy due to risk of bradycardia. Caution client regarding the risk of dizziness. Advise client and caregiver to notify health care provider if nausea, vomiting, diarrhea, or changes in color of stool occur or if new symptoms occur. Administer between meals; may be given with meals for GI symptoms. Due to risk of dizziness, assist with ambulation during the beginning of therapy. If drug overdose occurs, withdraw drug, administer tertiary anticholinergics, provide supportive care.

Education: Advise client and / or family that dosage may be adjusted to response no more than q 6 weeks. Instruct to report undesirable effects such as nausea, vomiting, sweating, or twitching which indicates toxicity. Instruct regarding the importance of not to increase or abruptly decrease dose due to the serious consequences that may result. Family and client need to understand that the drug is not a cure; it only relieves symptoms. Recommend taking drug in the evening just before going to bed.

Evaluation: Client will experience decrease in confusion, improved mood.

"A RICE PT"

A dminister in evening just prior to bedtime

R ifampin may result in drug/drug interactions

I ndicated for Alzheimer's

C aution for the "dreaded 'd's'": dizziness, drowsiness, depression, diarrhea, deep muscle cramps

E levation in acetylcholine

P ulse may become bradycardia

T ake without regard to food

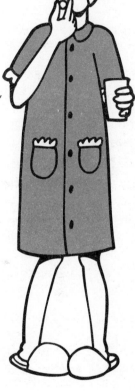

©2005 I CAN Publishing, Inc.

The client with Alzheimer's may need this medication. In early stages they may be very NICE. Later on, they may misinterpret their pill for a grain of RICE. "A RICE PT" will help you remember this Anti-Alzheimer's agent. Also remember "RICE" rhymes with "NICE".

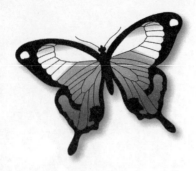

The Master sees things as they are, without trying to control them. She lets them go their own way, and resides at the center of the circle.

LAO-TZU
Tao-te-Ching

Reproductive and Women's Health-Related Agents

OXYTOCINS

Action: Stimulates contraction of uterine muscle fibers.

Indications: Pitocin—Induction of labor contractions; Ergotrate/Methergine (E/M)—Control uterine atony after delivery of placenta.

Warnings: Cephalopelvic disproportion, fetal distress, anticipated nonvaginal delivery. E/M—hypertension, preeclampsia, history of CVAs.

Undesirable Effects: Pitocin—Nausea/vomiting; hypertension, cardiac arrhythmias; uterine hypertonicity, fetal bradycardia; water intoxication with convulsions and coma. E/M: Most frequent: nausea/vomiting; Less frequent: HTN, dizziness.

Other Specific Information: Use cautiously with dopamine, vasoconstrictors, and regional anesthetics.

Interventions: Baseline and ongoing maternal HR and BP, uterine activity, and fetal heart rate (FHR). Monitor I & O every 2 hrs. Maintain client in sitting or left lateral recumbent position. Be alert for signs of uterine rupture (very infrequent), which include decreased or absent FHR, sudden increased pain, absent contractions, hemorrhage, and the rapid development of hypovolemic shock. Pitocin—IV administration under continuous observation. No bolus injection. Use infusion pump.

Education: Ergotrate—Instruct client to avoid smoking. Caution about exposure to cold. Alert client that discomfort may result form ergonovine-related contractions. Instruct about appropriate nonpharmacologic methods to decrease discomfort.

Evaluation: Positive uterine response; control of postpartum hemorrhage.

Drugs: ergonovine (Ergotrate); methylergonovine (Methergine); oxytocin (Pitocin, Syntocinon)

PITOCIN

Pressure is elevated

Intoxication with water

Tetanic contractions

Oxygen decrease in fetus

Cardiac arrhythmia

Irregularity in fetal heart rate

Nausea and vomiting

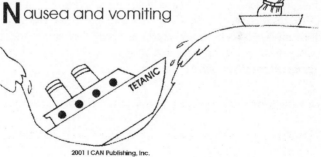

2001 I CAN Publishing, Inc.

Oxytocin "squeezes" and contracts the uterus to initiate labor and stop hemorrage after delivery.

MAGNESIUM SULFATE

Action: Reduces striated muscle contractions due to the depressant effect on the CNS. Blocks neuromuscular transmission.

Indications: Control of convulsions in preeclampsia or eclampsia.

Warnings: Do not give 2 hours preceding delivery because of risk of magnesium toxicity in neonate. Heart block, significant cardiac damage, or renal failure.

Undesirable Effects: Weakness, dizziness. Magnesium intoxication—flushing, sweating, hypotension, ↓ reflexes (patellar reflex is an indication regarding the depression of the CNS), ↓ respirations, flaccid paralysis, hypothermia, circulatory collapse, cardiac and CNS depression.

Other Specific Information: Neuromuscular blockade can be produced by neuromuscular agents such as gallamine, metocurine iodide, pancuronium, vecuronium.

Interventions: Monitor serum levels. Normal serum magnesium concentrations are 1.6 to 2.6 mEq/L. Monitor knee jerk reflex before repeated parenteral administration; maintain urine output at a level of 100 ml every 4 hours during parenteral administration. Antidote is calcium gluconate.

Education: Advise client to report undesirable effects such as sweating, flushing, muscle tremors, twitching, or inability to move extremities.

Evaluation: Convulsions will be controlled or prevented.

Drug: Magnesium Sulfate

A ROAD BLOCK TO PIH AND SEIZURES

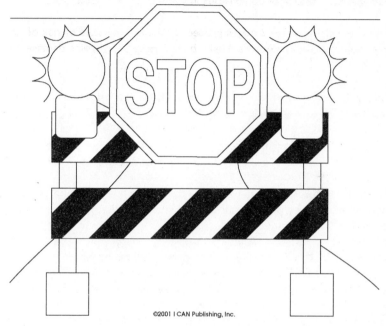

©2001 I CAN Publishing, Inc.

Magnesium sulfate, a CNS depressant, reduces or "stops" convulsions in the OB client.

Mag Sulfate

(sung to the tune of "Achy, Breaky Heart")

Decreased BP
Decreased Pee Pee
These are toxic signs of mag sulfate.
Drop in respiratory rate,
Patellar reflex there ain't,
Give antidote calcium gluconate!

(One more time)

BIOPHOSPHONATES

Action: Inhibits normal and abnormal bone resorption, without reducing mineralization.

Indications: Osteoporosis, Paget's disease.

Warnings: Hypersensitivity; renal dysfunction; concurrent use of hormone replacement. Gastrointestinal diseases; pregnancy/lactation.

Undesirable Effects: Headache; abdominal pain (most frequent): nausea, abdominal distension, constipation/diarrhea, flatulence, heartburn; muscle pain. Overdosage may result in GI disturbances.

Other Specific Information: Food, beverages, and dietary supplements may interfere with absorption. IV ranitidine may ↑ level.

Interventions: Baseline and periodical bone density studies and calcium levels. Monitor electrolytes. Calcium and vitamin D deficiency must be corrected prior to therapy.

Education: Instruct regarding the importance of taking with 6–8 oz of water, first thing in the morning and at least 30 minutes prior to first beverage, food, or medication of the day. Do not lie down for at least 30 minutes after taking medication to reduce risk of esophageal irritation. Advise client to participate in supportive lifestyle changes, such as stopping smoking, no alcohol, regular weight-bearing exercises. Discontinue and notify provider if chest pain occurs.

Evaluation: The client will reflect a decrease in the progression of osteoporosis as evidenced by the bone density studies and calcium levels.

Drug: alendronate (Fosamax), risedronate (Actonel)

JOSEPHINE BONE-A-PART

B one mass rebuilds

O nly take with full glass of water, no food

N ausea—never lie down after taking

E sophageal irritation

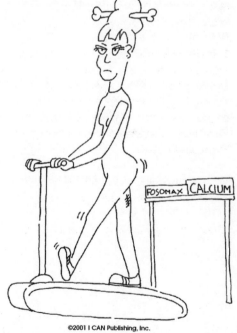

©2001 I CAN Publishing, Inc.

SELECTIVE ESTROGEN RECEPTOR MODULATOR (SERM)

Action: Has estrogen like effect on bone and lipid metabolism. Reduces resorption of bone and decreases overall bone turnover. Does not turn on breast or uterine receptors, (decreased risk of endometrial cancer).

Indications: Prevention of osteoporosis in postmenopausal women.

Warning: Pregnancy, blood clots.

Undesirable Effects: Hot flashes, leg cramps, infection. Rare: blood clots in the veins.

Other Specific Information: No increased risk of breast cancer and may be used in women with breast cancer.

Interventions: Discontinue 72 hours before and during prolonged immobilization; resume when fully ambulatory.

Education: Advise that medication may increase the risk of blood clots especially if there is a past history of clots in the legs, lungs, or eyes. May be taken with or without food at any time of the day. Avoid use with estrogen. Recommend that client also take a calcium supplement, vitamin D, stop smoking, and decrease alcohol intake.

Evaluation: Client's bone density studies will improve.

Drug: raloxifene (Evista)

SERM

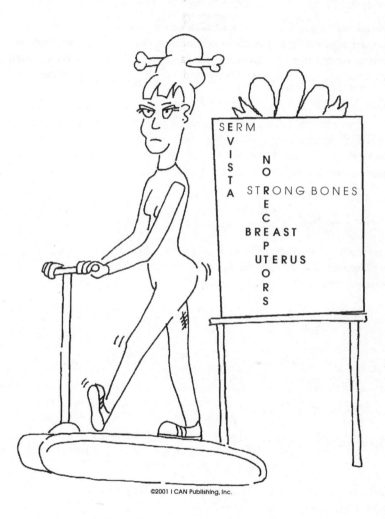

©2001 I CAN Publishing, Inc.

"SERM" is a gift to Josephine whose bones are coming "apart". **Selective Estrogen Receptor Modulators** are used to prevent osteoporosis in postmenopausal women. These drugs do not turn on breast or uterine receptors. The benefit "gift" is there is no increased risk of breast or endometrial cancer.

ESTROGEN

Action: Development and maintenance for adequate functioning of female reproductive system; affects release of pituitary gonadotropins; promotes adequate use in bone structures.

Indications: Moderate to severe vasomotor symptoms associated with menopause; postpartal breast engorgement, hormonal replacement therapy; prevention of osteoporosis and cardiovascular disease.

Warnings: Breast or reproductive cancer; estrogen dependent neoplasm; undiagnosed abnormal genital bleeding; thromboembolic disorders.

Undesirable Effects: Nausea, vomiting; headaches; breast tenderness; fluid retention, hypertension; leg cramps; break through bleeding; photosensitivity. Breast cancer, endometrial cancer. Gall bladder disease; mental depression; breast tenderness; change in libido; changes in vaginal bleeding pattern and alteration in bleeding and flow.

Other Specific Information: May ↓ effects of anticoagulant, oral hypoglycemic. ↓ effects with anticonvulsants, barbiturates, rifampin. Antibiotics ↓ the effects of estrogen. Toxicity with tricyclic antidepressants. ↑ effects of corticosteroids.

Interventions: Monitor blood pressure, weight, and serum glucose if client is a diabetic. Hepatic function studies should be done every 6 to 12 months for clients with hepatic dysfunction. Use lowest effective dose.

Education: Counsel client of childbearing age to use effective contraceptive method. Estrogens may cause congenital defects. Withdrawal bleeding may occur. Advise client to report severe headache, abdominal pain or mass, vomiting, breasts lumps, dizziness, fainting, shortness of breath, blurred vision, or break through bleeding. Teach client self breast examination. Explain cyclic manner in which drug is usually administered. Instruct how to use the ordered form: oral, intravaginal, transdermal. Provide with package insert for drug to inform client how to safely use the med and specific warning signs to report. Warn against cigarette smoking and sun tanning. Instruct to report positive urine or blood sugar tests. If taking conjugated or esterified estrogens for osteoporosis prophylaxis, advise to increase the intake of calcium and vitamin D and to participate in regular weight-bearing exercises. Inform client regarding the importance of annual PAP smears, mammograms, and cholesterol series.

Evaluation: Client will demonstrate an improvement in the condition for which the medication was given without any undesirable effects.

Drugs: *Esterified estrogens:* (Estratab, Estratest, Menest); estradiol (Climara, Estrace, Estrace Vaginal Cream, Estraderm, Vivelle); estradiol cypionate (depGynogen, Depo-Estradiol, Dura-Estrin, E-Cypionate, Estro-Cyp, Estrofem, Estroject-LA); estradiol valerate (Delestrogen, Dioval 40, Dioval XX, Duragen-20, Duragen-40, Estra-L 40, Feminate, Femogex, Gynogen L.A., Menaval, Valergen-10, Valergen-20, Valergen-40); *Conjugated estrogens:* (Premarin, Premarin Intravenous, Premphase, Prempro)

"ESTER" ESTROGEN

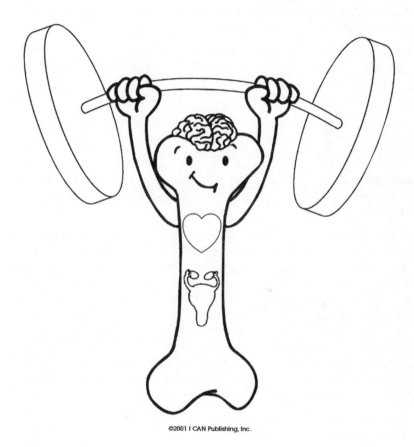

©2001 I CAN Publishing, Inc.

"Ester" Estrogen builds strength in bones (reducing bone loss) and protects the heart from cardiac disease. Estrogen also has been linked to the prevention of Alzheimer's. Estrogen helps maintain the functioning of the female reproductive system.

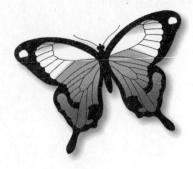

The willingness to accept responsibility for one's own life—is the source from which self respect springs.

John Didion

Vitamins, Minerals, and Electrolytes

VITAMIN: PYRIDOXINE

Action: A coenzyme necessary for many metabolic functions affecting carbohydrate, lipid, and protein utilization in the body.

Indications: Pyridoxine deficiency.

Warnings: Pregnancy. IV therapy in cardiac clients.

Undesirable Effects: Rare. Occasional stinging at IM injection site.

Other Specific Information: Pyridoxine decreases effect of levodopa and can lead to serious toxic effects. Isoniazid (INH) may antagonize pyridoxine (may cause anemia/peripheral neuritis).

Interventions: Monitor for improvement of nervous system abnormalities (anxiety, depression, insomnia, peripheral numbness, and tremors) and skin lesions (glossitis, seborrhea like lesions around eyes, mouth, nose).

Education: Discomfort may occur at IM site. Foods rich in pyridoxine include avocado, bananas, bran, eggs, hazelnuts, legumes, organ meats, shrimp, tuna, wheat germ.

Evaluation: The client will maintain an appropriate intake of pyridoxine, intact mucous membranes and skin, and normal mental and neurologic status.

Drug: pyridoxine (vitamin B_6)

B$_6$

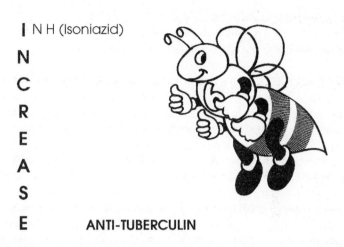

I N H (Isoniazid)
N
C
R
E
A
S
E

ANTI-TUBERCULIN

L evadopa
O
W
E
R

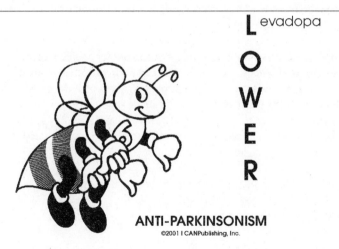

ANTI-PARKINSONISM
©2001 I CANPublishing, Inc.

Our "B$_6$" is telling you that, with his thumbs up, B$_6$ should be increased when taking INH.

"B$_6$"'s thumbs down with Levadopa. B$_6$ should be lowered to prevent toxicity.

FOLIC ACID
(Vitamin B9)

Action: Stimulates production of red and white blood cells and platelets. This is essential for nucleoprotein synthesis and the maintenance of normal erythropoiesis.

Indications: Megaloblastic, macrocytic anemia associated with pregnancy, infancy, childhood, inadequate dietary intake.

Warnings: Anemias (pernicious, aplastic, normocytic, refractory).

Undesirable Effects: Allergic hypersensitivity occurs rarely with parenteral form. Oral folic acid is nontoxic.

Other Specific Information: May decrease effects of hydantoin anticonvulsants. Analgesics, anticonvulsants, carbamazepine, estrogens may increase folic acid requirements. Antacids, cholestyramine may decrease absorption. Methotrexate, triamterene, trimethoprim may antagonize effects. May decrease vitamin B12 concentration.

Interventions: Pernicious anemia should be ruled out by Schilling test and vitamin B 12 blood level before therapy is initiated (may produce irreversible neurologic damage). Resistance to treatment may occur if decreased hematopoiesis, alcoholism, antimetabolic drugs or deficiency of vitamin B6, B12, or E is evident. Evaluate for improvement of vitamin deficiency such as: improved sense of well-being, relief from iron deficiency symptoms (fatigue, shortness of breath, sore tongue, headache, pallor).

Education: Folic acid should only be taken as prescribed. Foods high in folic acid should be encouraged such as fruits, vegetables, and organ meats. Hives or rash should be reported to provider of care immediately.

Evaluation: Client will present with a normal folic acid with no symptoms of anemia.

Drug: Folic Acid (Vitamin B9)

FOLIC ACID

F ood—bran, yeast, dried beans, nuts, fruits, fresh vegetables, asparagus

Gr **O** wth and production of erythrocytes

L iver disease, alcoholism, renal disease, pregnancy—issues

I nteraction—lowers metabolosm with anticonvulsants

C holestyramine may decrease absorption of folic acid

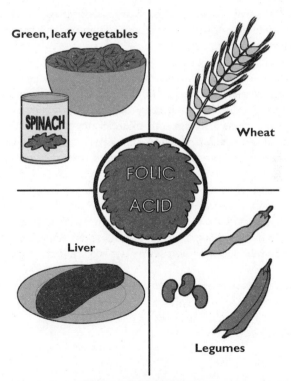

Green, leafy vegetables

SPINACH

Wheat

Liver

Legumes

©2005 I CAN Publishing, Inc.

VITAMIN B12

Action: Coenzyme for metabolic functions (fat, carbohydrate metabolism, protein synthesis). Necessary for growth, cell replication, hematopoiesis, and myelin synthesis.

Indication: Prophylaxis, treatment of pernicious anemia, vitamin B12 deficiency, thyrotoxicosis, hemorrhage, and renal and/or hepatic disease.

Warnings: History of allergy to cobalamin, folate deficient anemia, hereditary optic nerve atrophy. Use cautiously if client has heart disease, history of gout, pulmonary disease, undiagnosed anemia.

Undesirable Effects: Occasional diarrhea, itching. Rare allergic reaction generally due to impurities in the preparation. May produce peripheral vascular thrombosis, hypokalemia, pulmonary edema, CHF.

Other Specific Information: Alcohol, colchicines may decrease absorption. Ascorbic acid may destroy vitamin B 12. Folic acid in large doses may decrease concentration.

Interventions: Assess for CHF, pulmonary edema, hypokalemia in clients with cardiac disease receiving SubQ/ IM therapy. Monitor potassium levels (3.5–5mEq / L), serum B 12 (200–800 mg/ml), rise in reticulocyte count (peaks in 5-8 days). Assess for reversal of deficiency symptoms: hyporeflexia, loss of positional sense, ataxia, fatigue, irritability, insomnia, anorexia, pallor, palpitation on exertion. Therapeutic response to treatment usually within 48 hours.

Education: Lifetime treatment may be imperative for clients with pernicious anemia. Instruct client to report symptoms of infection. Encourage foods rich in vitamin B 12 such as organ meats, clams, herring, oysters, red snapper, muscle meats, fermented cheese, egg yolks, and dairy products.

Evaluation: The client will be asymptomatic of clinical signs of a low vitamin B 12.

Drug: cyanocobalamin (vitamin B 12)

VITAMIN B12

YES:

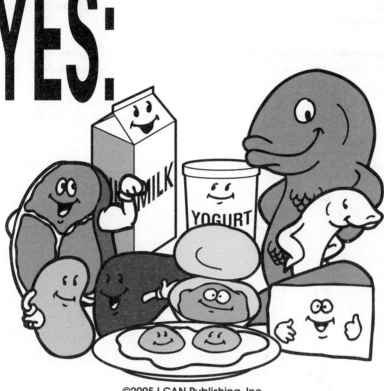

©2005 I CAN Publishing, Inc.

NO Ascorbic Acid
High Doses of B 9
(Folic Acid)

Foods at the top of this image are high in vitamin B12 and should be encouraged to be eaten. Ascorbic acid and high doses of folic acid may decrease or destroy vitamin B12.

VITAMIN K
(AquaMethyton)

Action: Needed for adequate blood clotting factors (II, VII, IX, X)

Indications: Vitamin K malabsorption, hypoprothrombinemia, prevention of hypoprothrombinemia caused by oral anticoagulants. Prevention of newborn complications with hemorrhagic disease.

Warnings: Hypersensitivity. Severe hepatic disease. Avoid IV use if possible. Give SQ or IM.

Undesirable Effects: Headache, nausea, hemolytic anemia, hyperbilirubinemia, rash.

Other Specific Information: Decreased action of oral anticoagulants. Decreased action of phytonadione when taken with cholestyramine, mineral oil.

Interventions: Assess for bleeding: emesis, stools, urine. Assess PT during treatment (2-sec. deviation from control time, bleeding time, and clotting time); monitor for bleeding, heart rate, and blood pressure.

Education: *Review foods high in vitamin K:* liver (beef), spinach, tomatoes, coffee, asparagus, broccoli, cabbage, lettuce, greens. Recommend not to take other supplements unless directed by provider of care. Instruct to avoid IM injections, use soft tooth brush, do not floss, use electric razor until coagulation defect has been corrected. Report signs of bleeding. Discuss the importance of frequent lab test to monitor coagulation factors.

Evaluate: Client will experience a decrease in bleeding tendencies, decreased PT, and decrease in the clotting time.

Drug: phytonadione (AquaMEPHYTON)

VITAMIN K

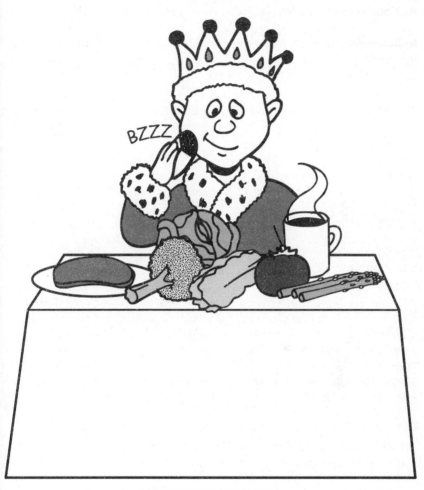

©2004 I CAN Publishing, Inc.

MINERAL: IRON

Action: Operates as an oxygen carrier in hemoglobin.

Indications: Prevents and treats iron deficiency anemia.

Warnings: Hemolytic anemia, peptic ulcer, ulcerative colitis.

Undesirable Effects: Nausea, vomiting, constipation, and abdominal cramps.

Other Specific Information: ↑ effect of iron with vitamin C; ↓ absorption with antacids, cimetidine. Coffee, tea, milk, eggs, whole grain breads and cereals ↓ iron absorption.

Interventions: Monitor RBC count, hemoglobin, hematocrit, iron level, and reticulocyte count. Administer IM injection by the Z-track method.

Education: Instruct to take drug between meals with at least 8 oz. of juice (vitamin C enhances absorption of iron) or water. Instruct client to take liquid iron with a straw. If GI distress is experienced, advise to take with food. Swallow whole tablet or capsule. Do not take drug within 1 hour of taking antacid or milk. Recommend increasing fluids, fiber, and exercise to decrease constipation. Instruct not to leave iron within reach of children. Review with client that treatment for anemia is generally < 6 months. Review diet high in iron such as liver, lean meats, legumes, green vegetables, and fruit. Stool may turn black or dark green.

Evaluation: The client will participate in activities with no fatigue or shortness of breath. The hemoglobin, hematocrit, reticulocyte count, and plasma iron values will remain in normal range.

Drugs: ferrous fumarate (Feostat, Ferrous fumarate); ferrous gluconate (Fergon, Ferralet); ferrous sulfate (Feosol, Fer-Iron)

IRON

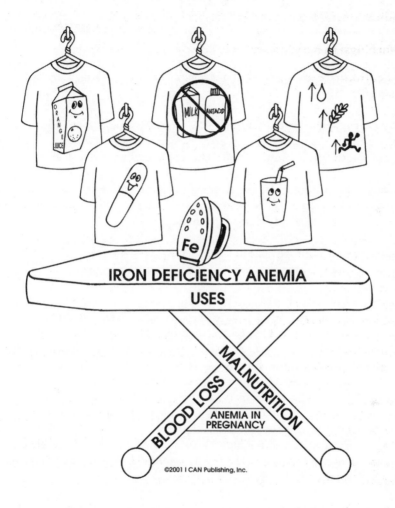

Iron improves iron deficiency anemia, anemia in pregnancy, malnutrition and blood loss.

When administering iron, the 5 hangers will assist you in remembering the priority teaching tips. Starting from left to right: take iron with vitamin C, swallow whole tablet or capsule (do not crush), do not take with milk or antacid, take liquid iron with a straw, and increase fluid, fiber and exercise.

ELECTOLYTE: POTASSIUM

Action: Necessary for many cellular metabolic processes; primary action is intracellular. Conducts nerve impulses; contracts cardiac, skeletal, smooth muscle. Maintains normal renal function.

Indications: Correct potassium deficiency. Strengthen cardiac and muscular activities.

Warnings: Addison's disease, cardiac/renal insufficiency, hyperkalemia, acidosis, burns, potassium-sparing diuretics, ACE inhibitors. Never push K CL. Always dilute. Solutions more diluted for peripheral vs. central line.

Undesirable Effects: Nausea, vomiting, diarrhea, abdominal discomfort, rash (rare), hyperkalemia manifested as cold skin, paresthesia of extremities, hypotension, confusion, cardiac arrhythmias.

Other Specific Information: ↑ serum potassium level with ACE inhibitors, potassium-sparing diuretics, and salt substitutes using potassium.

Interventions: Monitor serum potassium level (therapeutic 3.5–5.0 mEq/L), vital signs, ECG, and signs of hyper or hypokalemia. Assess signs of digitalis toxicity. Give IV infusions as diulte solution infuses slowly. Observe IV site for infiltration so tissue necrosis will not occur. **Potassium should never be given as an IV bolus or push.** Potassium CANNOT be given IM. Monitor urine output. 80–90% of potassium is excreted in the urine.

Education: Recommend client to have serum potassium level checked at regular intervals. Instruct to take oral preparation with at least 6–8 oz. of water or juice and at mealtime. Medical follow-up to the health related problem and medication is important. Review foods rich in potassium (i.e., bananas, canteloupes, oranges, raisins, potatoes).

Evaluation: Client's potassium level will remain in normal range.

Drugs: potassium acetate (Potassium acetate); potassium chloride (Kaochlor, K-Dur, K-Lor, Klotrix, K-Lyte/Cl, Slow-K); potassium gluconate (Kaon)

POTASSIUM

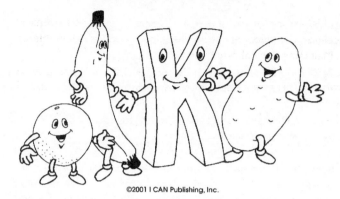

©2001 I CAN Publishing, Inc.

P otassium sparing diuretics—monitor K$^+$

O utput—monitor closely

T ake with food

A ce Inhibitors—monitor K$^+$

S igns of digitalis toxicity if K$^+$ is ↓

S erum potassium level —3.5–5.0 mEq/L

I V postassium ▽HIGH ALERT

U ndesirable Effects: N/V, cardiac arrhythmias

M edical follow-up

SUPPLEMENT: CALCIUM

Action: Promotes strong bones and teeth growth.

Indications: Prevents osteoporosis. Corrects calcium deficiency. Hyperacidity associated with peptic ulcer disease.

Warnings: Hypercalcemia, digitalis toxicity, renal calculi, ventricular fibrillation, renal, cardiac, or respiratory disorders.

Undesirable Effects: Nausea, vomiting, constipation; pain, headache; slowed heart rate; peripheral vasodilation.

Other Specific Information: Decreased effect of verapamil and decreased serum levels of oral tetracyclines, salicylates, and iron salts. Decreased absorption of oral calcium when taken with oxalic acid (found in rhubarb and spinach), phytic acid (bran and whole cereals), and phosphorus (milk and dairy products).

Interventions: Observe for anorexia, nausea, vomiting, and headache. Monitor serum calcium. Record consistency of stools.

Education: Instruct to take oral calcium supplements with food. Administer calcium carbonate antacid 1 and 3 hours after meals and at bedtime. Take other oral medications at least 1–2 hrs after calcium carbonate. Chew antacid tablets completely prior to swallowing; drink 1 full glass of water or milk after swallowing tablet. If taking suspension, shake and take with a small amount of water. Review foods high in calcium; protein and vitamin D are necessary to enhance calcium absorption. Avoid overuse of antacids and laxatives. For clients who are treating osteoporosis, review the importance of engaging in weight bearing exercises. Recommend that client discuss with provider of care about the pros and cons of estrogen supplement.

Evaluation: The calcium level will be within normal limits, and client will experience no signs of hypo or hypercalcemia. If being treated for osteoporosis, the bone density will be normal.

Drugs: calcium carbonate (Caltrate, Chooz, Equilet, OsCAL, Oystercal, Tums)

CALCIUM

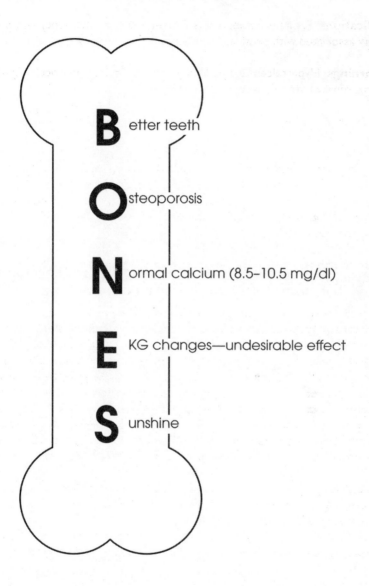

Better teeth

Osteoporosis

Normal calcium (8.5–10.5 mg/dl)

EKG changes—undesirable effect

Sunshine

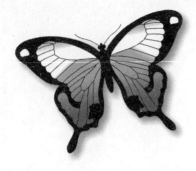

A life spent making mistakes is not only more honorable, but more useful than a life spent doing nothing.

George Bernard Shaw

Complementary Agents

NOTE: As a pharmacist, I would caution against the use of these agents. The manufacturers of these agents are not required to follow the Good Manufacturing Practice Act as pharmaceutical manufacturers are required. The integrity of these agents cannot be guaranteed. Users are at an increased risk for drug interactions if taking these agents with prescription medications. Buyer beware!

—Nicole Blackwelder, PharmD.

Editors' Note: We have included these agents because of the increasing use of complementary agents by clients. Also, complementary agents are included on the NCLEX-RN® exam.

—Loretta and Sylvia

COENZYME Q10

Action: Co-Q10 has antioxidant and membrane-stabilizing properties. Co-Q10 is a free radical scavenger; protects cell membranes and DNA from oxidative damage. It is found in all human cells. Tissue is protected from ischemic cellular damage.

Indications: Allergies, asthma, respiratory disease; Alzheimer's, and schizophrenia. Gives energy to the heart especially in congestive heart failure.

Warnings: Hypersensitivity to Co-Q10.

Undesirable Effects: Anorexia, nausea, diarrhea, epigastric discomfort.

Other Specific Information: Oral antidiabetic agents may ↓ effectiveness of Co-Q10. Co-Q10 may ↓ response to warfarin.

Interventions: Cardiovascular assessment should be ongoing. Coenzyme Q 10 is oil soluble and is best absorbed when taken with oily or fatty foods, such as fish.

Education: Co-Q10 is perishable and deteriorates in temperatures above 115°F; a liquid form or oil form is preferable. Vitamin E helps preserve this coenzyme. Foods highest in vitamin E include mackerel, salmon and sardines; other foods include peanuts, spinach, and beef. Caution client not to perform intense exercise during Co-Q10 therapy due to potential damage of ischemic tissue. Instruct client with heart failure to inform health care provider of any clinical changes.

Evaluation: Client will have no signs of heart failure such as peripheral edema, hepatosplenomegaly, jugular vein distention, S_3, and basilar crackles. The client will have a normal sinus rhythm on the ECG and will have an increased sense of well being. Client will have a decrease in the symptoms for which the herb was administered.

Drugs: Adelir, Co-Q10, Heartcin, Inokiton, Neuquinone, Taidecanone, Ubiquinone, Udekinon

COENZYME Q10

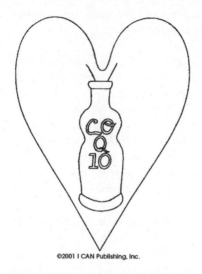

©2001 I CAN Publishing, Inc.

E —Vitamin helps preserve Co-Q10

N ausea, vomiting, anorexia—U E

al**Z** heimer's, schizophrenia; CHF—indications

Y ES, it has ANTI-AGING effects

M ackeral, Salmon, and Sardines— ↑in vitamin E

E ffectiveness of Co-Q10 is ↓with oral antidiabetics

The energy for the heart is coming from the "Coke™ Co-Q10 bottle". "ENZYME" will help recall some key facts.

ECHINACEA

Action: Stimulates phagocytosis; increases mobility of leukocytes; increases respiratory cellular activity. This results in an increased immune, antiseptic, antiviral, immunostimulant, anti-inflammatory, and antibacterial effect. Has peripheral vasodilator properties.

Indications: Sore throat, colds, flu; low immune status; cancer. External ointments used for burns, ulcerations, eczema, herpes simplex, psoriasis, and wounds that heal poorly. Reduces recurrence of Candida albicans and decreases the growth of Trichomonas vaginalis.

Warnings: Externally, none known. Internally, progressive systemic diseases such as tuberculosis, multiple sclerosis, HIV (including AIDS), collagen diseases, or other autoimmune diseases. Alcoholics and clients with liver disease. Pregnancy, breastfeeding, children.

Undesirable Effects: Allergies may occur if client is allergic to plants in the daisy family.

Other Specific Information: Do not administer with immunosuppressants or hepatotoxic drugs. Many tinctures contain significant amount of alcohol, so avoid disulfiram or metronidazole.

Interventions: Monitor WBCs, vital signs, and breath sounds (respiratory diseases).

Education: Instruct client that herb should not be used longer than 8 weeks; 10–14 days of therapy is probably sufficient. If illness does not resolve after taking the herb, advise to notify provider.

Evaluation: WBCs will return to normal range. Temperature will return to normal range, and client will have a decrease in the symptoms for which the herb was administered.

Drugs: Coneflower Extract, Echinacea, Echinacea Angustifolia Herb, Echinacea Fresh Freeze-Dried, Echinacea Glycerite, Echinacea Herb, Echinacea Herbal Comfort Lozenges, Echinacea Purpurea

ECHINACEA

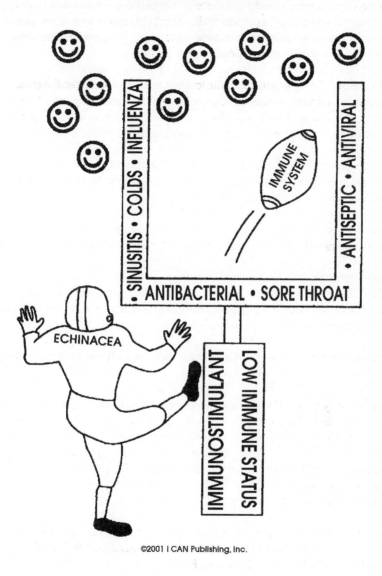

©2001 I CAN Publishing, Inc.

Echinacea is giving a powerful boost to the immune system so colds, flu, sore throats will heal quickly and smiles will return.

EVENING PRIMROSE

Action: The evening primrose oil stems from essential fatty acids that are crucial as structural elements for cells and as precursors of synthesis of prostaglandins. Linoleic acid is not manufactured by the body and must be provided through diet. The body relies on the metabolic conversion of linoleic acid (LA) to gamma linoleic acid (GLA). A deficiency in this process results in diabetes, cancer, CV disease, hypercholesterolemia, etc. This herb contains the highest amount of GLA of any food substance.

Indications: Rheumatoid arthritis, PMS, menopause, and diabetic neuropathy.

Warnings: Pregnancy, breast cancer, schizophrenia, or clients taking epileptogenic medications such as phenothiazines.

Undesirable Effects: Abdominal discomfort, nausea, headache, rash, immunosuppression may occur after use of GLA for > 1 yr.

Other Specific Information: Phenothiazines may ↑ risk of seizures.

Interventions: Use Oil of Evening Primrose for the best source of gamma linoleic acid.

Education: Instruct women with breast cancer or clients with a seizure disorder not to use this herb.

Evaluation: The client's symptoms will improve based on the therapeutic reason for taking the herb.

Drugs: Efamol, Epogram, Evening Primrose Oil, Mega Primrose Oil, My Favorite Evening Primrose Oil, Primrose Power

EVENING PRIMROSE

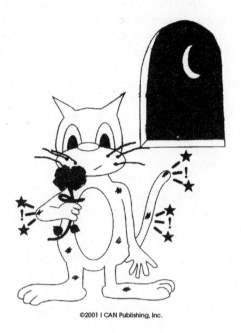

©2001 I CAN Publishing, Inc.

R heumatoid athritis, PMS, menopause: indications

O il of Evening Primrose—best source of GLA

S eizures ↑ risk if herb is taken with phenothiazines

E ducation—don't use if client has a history of
    breast cancer or seizures

Kat smells the primrose oil to enhance her amorous activities for the night. Of course if she were having hot flashes, the evening primrose would reduce those right along with the pain she may be having from rheumatoid arthritis.

FEVERFEW

Actions: Inhibits synthesis of prostaglandins and leukotrienes. Inhibits secretion of serotonin from platelet granules. These substances are known to increase in the brain during the early phase of migraine attack.

Indications: Migraine headaches, arthritis, fever, and menstrual disorders.

Warnings: Pregnancy or breast-feeding.

Undesirable Effects: Occasional mouth ulceration or gastric disturbance, dry and sore tongue, swollen lips, abdominal pain, vomiting, diarrhea, and flatulence. Post-feverfew syndrome (withdrawal syndrome characterized by moderate to severe pain and joint and muscle stiffness).

Other Specific Information: Use caution with anticoagulants; may ↑ bleeding.

Interventions: Recommend avoiding chewing the leaves since they can cause mouth ulcers.

Education: Discuss proper oral hygiene due to the risk of mouth ulcerations. Discuss the importance of reporting undesirable effects to provider. Even though feverfew is given for pain, the user can still operate heavy machinery. Treatment for at least a few months is recommended. Instruct client not to withdraw the herb abruptly.

Evaluation: Client's temperature will return to normal range and pain will subside.

Drugs: Feverfew, Feverfew Glyc, Feverfew Power

MYRA MIGRAINE

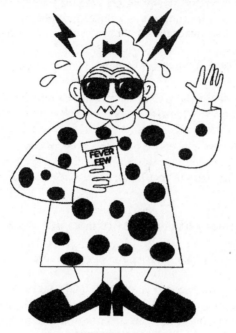

©2001 I CAN Publishing, Inc.

M ay cause mouth ulcers

Y ou can't use during pregnancy

R educes pain

A nticoagulants may cause bleeding

Myra Migraine is holding her jar of Feverfew leaves that reduce the pain of her headaches and photophobia. It has also stimulated Myra's appetite and her dress size is about to outgrow her "big hair".

GARLIC

Action: Inhibits platelet aggregation (blood thinner). Decreases lipids and has antitumor effects.   Lowers total serum cholesterol, triglycerides, and low-density lipoprotein (LDL), while increasing high-density lipoprotein (HDL). Garlic also has antitumor and antimicrobial effects.

Indications: Lowers high blood pressure and serum lipid levels; aids in the treatment of arteriosclerosis; yeast or wound infections; colds and flu.

Warnings: Hypersensitivity, peptic ulcer or reflux disease. Pregnant women due to oxytocic effects.

Undesirable Effects: The entire body can smell of garlic; diaphoresis; hypothyroidism; irritation of mouth, esophagus, or stomach; nausea / vomiting. Chronic use may lead to decreased hemoglobin production and lysis of RBCs.

Other Specific Information: Anticoagulants may ↑ risk of bleeding.

Interventions: Monitor CBC if client taking high-dose or long-term garlic.

Education: Aged garlic extract is desirable. May give the entire body a garlic odor. Odorless garlic supplements are available. Instruct client to watch for signs of bleeding (bleeding gums, bruising, petechiae) if taking with hemostatic agents.

Evaluation: The client will have a decrease in BP, lipid levels, or clinical symptoms for which the garlic was administered.

Drugs: Garlic, Garlic-Power, Garlique, Kwai, Kyolic, Odorless Garlic Tablets, One a Day Garlic, Sapec

GARLIC

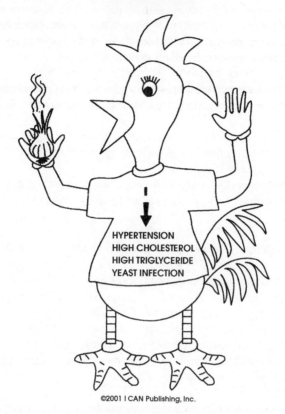

HYPERTENSION
HIGH CHOLESTEROL
HIGH TRIGLYCERIDE
YEAST INFECTION

©2001 I CAN Publishing, Inc.

O bserve for bleeding if taking anticoagulants

D oes also have antitumor and antimicrobial effects

O dorless garlic supplements are available

R eevaluate BP and lab reports

Garlic Chicken is much improved from her high cholesterol, triglycerides and high blood pressure. Garlic also helps her yeast infection.

GINGER

Action: Reduces spasms and cramps in the colon. A strong antioxidant and effective antimicrobial agent for sores and wounds. Inhibits platelet aggregation induced by ADP and epinephrine. Other studies have suggested that components in ginger may be gastroprotective against various chemical insults and stressors. It is postulated to be from increased mucosal resistance and potentiation of the defensive mechanism against chemicals or alterations in prostaglandins, providing more protective effects.

Indications: Nausea, motion sickness, indigestion, inflammation.

Warnings: *Pregnant clients:* Use only under medical supervision in clients receiving anticoagulants because it may affect bleeding time by inhibiting platelet function.

Undesirable Effects: Possible CNS depression or arrhythmias with overdose.

Other Specific Information: Anticoagulants may enhance risk of bleeding.

Interventions: Monitor for undesirable effects. Evaluate for signs of bleeding.

Education: Advise the female client to avoid use of ginger during pregnancy. Instruct client to watch for signs of bleeding when taking ginger. Explain that no consensus exists with respect to the exact dose.

Evaluation: Client will experience therapeutic results from the ginger (i.e., nausea will subside, indigestion will subside, etc.)

Drugs: Cayenne Ginger, Gingerall, Ginger Peppermint Combo, Ginger Power, Ginger Trips

GINGER

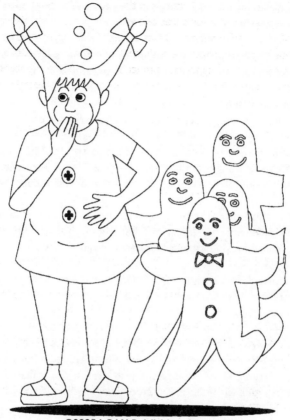

©2005 I CAN Publishing, Inc.

G ive to reduce spasms in colon

I ncreased risk of bleeding with anticoagulants

N ausea—use

Gingerbread men rush to the rescue of nausea and vomiting.

GINKGO BILOBA

Action: The herb produces arterial and venous vasoactive changes that increase the tissue perfusion and cerebral blood flow. Stimulates prostaglandin biosynthesis. Acts as an anti-oxidant.

Indications: Memory loss; early stages of Alzheimer's disease; poor circulation to extremities, intermittent claudication; antioxidant.

Warnings: Hypersensitivity; pregnancy, children; hemophilia or bleeding disorders; clients taking anticoagulants or antiplatelet agents.

Undesirable Effects: These are rare. Mild gastrointestinal upset in less than 1% of clients. Long-term use has been linked with rare occurrences of spontaneous subdural hematoma, intracerebral or intraocular hemorrhage.

Other Specific Information: Cigarette smoking and/or use of platelet-aggregation inhibitors may ↑ risk of subarachnoid hemorrhage. May interact with carbemazepine, phenobarbital, phenytoin, and TCAs.

Interventions: Administration for at least 2 weeks recommended. Children and adults taking medicinal doses should be seen by a qualified health care provider.

Education: Stay within recommended dosage and duration. Advise to take no aspirin or NSAIDs or alcohol; report unusual bleeding or bruising. Keep out of reach from children due to the potential risk of seizures with ingestion. Avoid contact with the fruit pulp or seed coats due to risk of dermatitis.

Evaluation: Substantial regression of major symptoms of chronic cerebral insufficiency including vertigo, senility, fatigue, lack of vigilance, and poor circulation to the limbs.

Drugs: Bioginkgo 24/6, Bioginkgo 27/7, Gincosan, Ginexin Remind, Ginkai, Ginkgoba, Ginkgo Go!, Ginkgold, Ginkgo Phytosome, Ginkgo Power, Ginkoba

GINKO

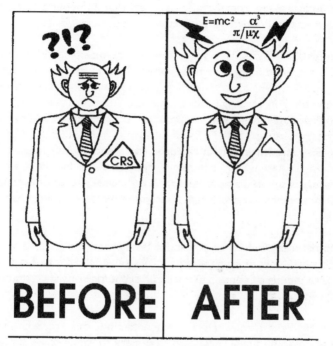

©2001 I CAN Publishing, Inc.

As indicated by the initials on his handkerchief, Gink **"can't remember shit!"** A few weeks on Ginko Biloba and he receives the benefits of increased memory and decreased depression. He can just feel the better blood flow through his brain and can now think like Einstein!

GINSENG

Action: Supports and enhances adrenal function, allowing for more consistent energy and better reaction to stress. Reduces cholesterol and triglycerides, decreases platelet adhesiveness and coagulation, and increases fibrinolysis. Antiarrhythmic effects have also been determined with ginseng similar to verapamil and amiodarone.

Indications: Improves stamina, concentration, and stress-resistance; adjunct in radiation and chemotherapy. Lowers blood glucose and cholesterol levels; and has antihypertensive effects.

Warnings: Cardiovascular disease, hyper / hypotension, diabetes, or clients receiving steroid therapy. Pregnancy, breast-feeding.

Undesirable Effects: High doses can cause jitters, headaches, and hypertension. Vaginal bleeding, skin eruptions, and pruritus have also been noted.

Other Specific Information: Antidiabetic agents should be used cautiously due to ginseng's hypoglycemic effect. MAO inhibitors given with ginseng may result in tremors, headache, and mania. Anticoagulants, aspirin, NSAIDs may inhibit blood clotting. Herb may interfere with digoxin's effects.

Interventions: Monitor for "Ginseng Abuse Syndrome" (i.e., nervousness, irritability, insomnia, morning diarrhea). This can occur if tea or coffee are taken with the herb. Monitor the diabetic client for signs and symptoms of hypoglycemia.

Education: Take 1 hour before eating. Vitamin C can interfere with absorption. Avoid caffeine. Take early in the day to reduce over stimulation. Generally up to 3 months is recommended. Advise a client with preexisting medical problems to be evaluated by the health care provider prior to taking ginseng. Review undesirable effects and report to provider of health care.

Evaluation: Client will experience an increase in energy and an improvement of symptoms for which ginseng was administered.

Drugs: Bio Star, Cimexon, Gincosan, Ginsana, Ginsatonic, Neo Ginsana

GINSENG

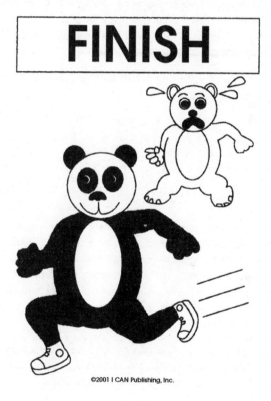

FINISH

©2001 I CAN Publishing, Inc.

GINSENG BEAR GETS TO THE FINISH LINE FIRST! He has taken his tonic that improves stamina and fights fatigue. Needless to say, the second bear in the race did not take his ginseng.

GOLDENSEAL

Action: Astringent, anti-inflammatory, oxytocic, antihemorrhagic, and laxative properties. Decreases the anticoagulant effects of heparin and acts as a cardiac stimulant. It increases coronary perfusion and inhibits cardiac activity. Antipyretic activity(greater than aspirin), antimuscarinic, antihistaminic, antitumor, antimicrobial, antihelmintic and hypotensive effects have also been documented.

Indications: GI disorders, gastritis, peptic ulceration, anorexia, postpartum hemorrhage, dysmenorrhea, eczema, pruritus, mouth ulcerations, otorrhoea, tinnitus, and conjunctivitis and as a wound antiseptic, diuretic, laxative, and anti-inflammatory agent.

Warnings: Clients with CV disease, particularly heart failure, arrhythmias, and during pregnancy.

Undesirable Effects: Asystole, bradycardia, CNS depression, contact dermatitis, diarrhea, GI cramping, heart block, leukocytosis, nausea, paresthesia, respiratory depression (with high doses), seizures, vomiting. Death may be caused by large alkaloid doses. Symptoms of overdose include GI upset, nervousness, depression, exaggerated reflexes, and convulsions that progress to respiratory paralysis and CV collapse.

Other Specific Information: Anticoagulants may reduce the beneficial effects of therapeutic anticoagulants. Antihypertensive agents may interfere or enhance hypotensive effects when taken with goldenseal or its extracts. Beta blockers, calcium channel blockers, digoxin may enhance or interfere with the cardiac effects of these drugs. Don't use together. CNS depressants (alcohol, benzodiazepines) may enhance sedative effects. Do not use with goldenseal.

Interventions: Monitor for signs of vitamin B deficiencies (megaloblastic anemia, peripheral neuropathy, seizures, cheilosis, glossitis, angular stomatitis, and infertility). Monitor for other undesirable effects.

Education: Recommend the client to avoid hazardous activities until CNS effects of the agent are known.

Evaluation: Client will experience therapeutic effects from the medication.

Drugs: Golden Seal Extract, Golden Seal Extract 4:1, Golden Seal Power, Golden Seal Root, Nu Veg Golden Seal Root, Nu Veg Golden Seal Herb

GOLDENSEAL

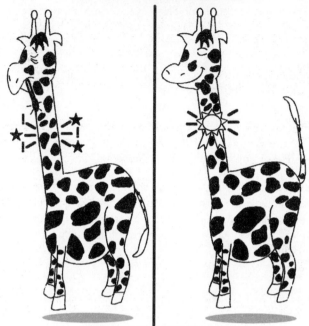

©2005 I CAN Publishing, Inc.

G I disorders and gastritis can benefit from this herb

O verdose—symptoms are GI upset, nervousness and seizures

L eukocytosis—undesirable effect

D o not administer anticoagulants, antihypertensive agents

E valuate for signs of vitamin B deficiency

N ot given to clients with CV disease

Gerry Giraffe has placed a golden seal on his infected throat and respiratory tract to help with his infection. His travel back to Africa will be improved since Goldenseal also treats traveler's diarrhea.

KAVA-KAVA

Action: The limbic system is inhibited by kavapyrones, an effect associated with suppression of emotional excitability and mood enhancement. Noted for promoting relaxation without loss of mental sharpness.

Indications: Anxiety disorders, stress, insomnia, muscle spasms, backache, neck ache, and pain from TMJ.

Warnings: Pregnant, breast-feeding, or children < 12. Use cautiously in clients with renal disease, neutropenia, or thrombocytopenia. Do not take if diagnosed with Parkinson's disease.

Undesirable Effects: Mild gastrointestinal disturbances; alterations in motor reflexes and judgment; visual disturbances. Dry, discolored flaking skin; reddened eyes (may be from cholesterol metabolism). Dopamine antagonism. ↓ patellar reflexes, pulmonary hypertension, and shortness of breath. ↓ bilirubin levels, plasma proteins, and urea. Weight loss. Long term use—↓ platelet and lymphocyte count.

Other Specific Information: When taken with kava these interactions can occur. Alprazolam may cause coma. Benzodiazepines, alcohol, and other CNS depressants ↑ sedative effects. Levodopa ↑ Parkinsonian symptoms. Pentobarbitol may have ↑ effects.

Interventions: Monitor for undesirable effects.

Education: Warn against using with medicines referred to in "Other Specific Information." Do not take for more than 3 months without provider advice due to significant undesirable effects. Instruct client to take with food.

Evaluation: Client will experience a decrease in anxiety and an improvement in peaceful sleep.

Drugs: Aigin, Antares, Ardeydystin, Cefkava, Kavasedon, Kavasporal, Kavatino, Laitan, Mosaro, Nervonocton N, Potter's Antigian Tablets, Viocava

KAVA-KAVA

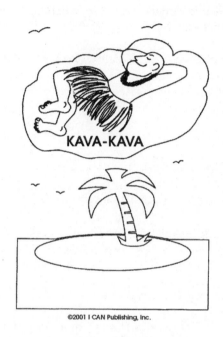

KAVA-KAVA

©2001 I CAN Publishing, Inc.

K ava interacts with CNS depressants

A dvise to take with food

V isual and mild GI disturbances: U E

A lprazolam given with Kava may cause a coma

Kava-Kava has been restless, nervous, anxious, and unable to sleep, but she is now floating on her cloud of calm. She will not be able to stay on her cloud for too long, because this herb also acts as a diuretic.

MILK THISTLE

Action: Hepatoprotective and antihepatotoxic actions over liver toxins. Silymarin, seeds from milk thistle, alters the outer liver membrane cell structure so that toxins cannot enter the cell. It also stimulates RNA polymerase A, which enhances ribosome protein synthesis and leads to activation of the regenerative capacity of the liver through cell development.

Indications: Alcoholic cirrhosis and hepatitis, antiinflammatory.

Warnings: Pregnant or breast-feeding clients. Caution with clients who have a hypersensitivity to plants belonging to the Asteraceae family.

Undesirable Effects: Mild laxative effect. Uterine and menstrual stimulation.

Other Specific Information: No interactions reported.

Interventions: Monitor liver function test results.

Education: Advise the client to consult with a medical professional in liver disease prior to starting this therapy. Report planned or suspected pregnancy. Instruct the client to report unusual symptoms immediately.

Evaluation: Client will experience therapeutic effects from the milk thistle.

Drugs: Beyond Milk Thistle, Milk Thistle Extract, Milk Thistle Phytosol, Milk Thistle Power, NU VEG Milk Thistle Power, Silymarin

MILK THISTLE

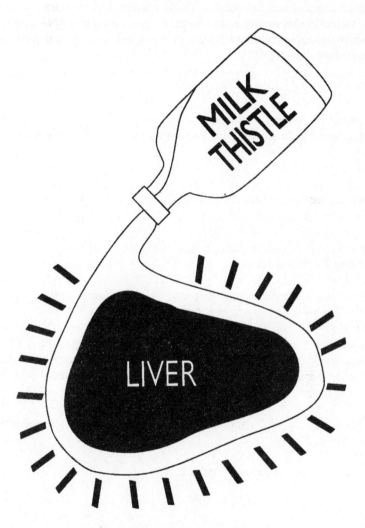

©2005 I CAN Publishing, Inc.

Milk Thistle alters the outer liver so that toxins cannot enter the liver cells.

SAW PALMETTO BERRY: SERENOA REPENS

Action: Lipidosterolic extract of S. repens (LSESR) appears to have an inhibitory effect on the binding of dihydrotestosterone (DHT) to androgen receptors in the prostate. LSESR also has an anti-inflammatory effect.

Indications: Benign prostate enlargement (BPH); may function as a mild diuretic.

Warnings: Pregnancy, breast-feeding, and women of childbearing age. Use cautiously in clients with medical problems other than BPH due to lack of data.

Undesirable Effects: Large amounts may cause diarrhea. In rare cases, stomach problems and headaches may occur. May create false-negative prostate-specific antigen (PSA) results.

Other Specific Information: ↑ side effects of estrogen or birth control pills. May ↓ iron absorption.

Interventions: Obtain a baseline prostate-specific antigen (PSA) before starting the herb since it can cause a false-negative PSA.

Education: Instruct client to take herb with AM and PM meal to ↓ GI effects. Client should use herb for BPH only after a diagnosis has been made and with the management of the provider of health care. Advise client to report any undesirable effects.

Evaluation: Client will experience a decrease in the symptoms for which the herb was taken.

Drugs: Permixon, Propalmex, Strogen

SAW PALMETTO

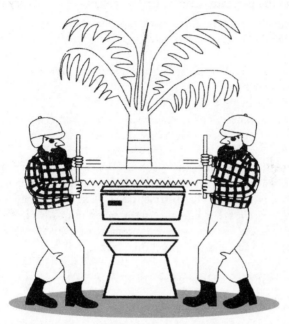

©2001 I CAN Publishing, Inc.

S tomach problems and headaches may occur

A lters PSA (prostate-specific antigen) test. May cause false negative

W atch for bloody urine

These two non-spring chicken men are sawing the toilet in half. They want to keep from spending their nights standing at the commode due to frequency of urination from enlarged prostate glands.

ST. JOHN'S WORT

Action: The exact mechanism has not been determined. Inhibits the stress-induced increase in corticotropin-releasing hormone, adrenocorticotropic hormone, and cortisol; increases the nocturnal melatonin levels. St. John's Wort has an antiviral activity.

Indications: Mild to moderate depression, insomnia, anxiety, and PMS symptoms; wound healing, insect bites.

Warnings: Clients taking prescription antidepressants. Pregnant or breast-feeding clients; children.

Undesirable Effects: Photosensitivity in people with fair skin. Dizziness, constipation, dry mouth, GI distress, restlessness.

Other Specific Information: Alcohol, MAO inhibitors, narcotics, OTC cold and flu medications, sympathomimetics, tyramine-containing foods may ↑ MAO inhibition activity. Paroxetine may ↑ sedative-hypnotic effects with the herb. Serotonin syndrome may occur when used with SSRIs or tricyclic antidepressants. Do not use with drugs that cause photosensitivity (i.e., sulfonamides, tetracyclines, antipsychotics, etc.).

Interventions: The client's depression should be evaluated by a health care provider.

Education: Use over a period of several weeks or months to obtain the desired effect. Best under supervision of health provider. Should not be used at the same time as prescription antidepressants. Avoid foods high in tyramine such as red wines, beer, aged cheese, glandular meats (liver), colas and chocolate. Teach to say out of the sun.

Evaluation: Client's communication and behavior will indicate an improvement of depression.

Drugs: Hypercalm, Hypericum, Kira, Mood Support, St. John's Wort, Nutri Zac, Tension Tamer

ST. JOHN'S WORT

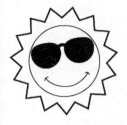

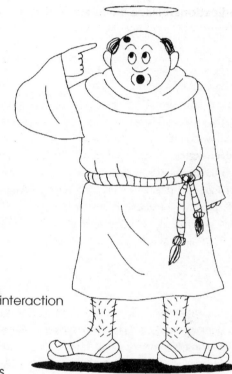

Watch the sun, Warfarin interaction

OK for stings and bites

Reduces viral infections

©2001 I CAN Publishing, Inc.

Taking MAOIs and SSRIs may cause serious U E

St. John's Wort on his head is making him anxious and unable to sleep. St. John's Wort calms the emotions and is used for depression.

ALPHABETICAL INDEX

B

Benzodiazepines 266, 267
(C-IV controlled substance):
alprazolam (Xanax)
chlordiazepoxide (Librium)
clonazepam (Klonopin)
clorazepate (Tranxene)
diazepam (Valium)
lorazepam (Ativan)
midazolam (Versed)
oxazepam (Serax)
Beta Adrenergic Blockers 56, 57
Cardioselective (Beta 1 receptors):
acebutolol (Sectral)
atenolol (Tenormin)
betaxolol (Kerlone)
bisoprolol (Zebeta)
esmolol (Brevibloc)
metoprolol (Lopressor, Toprol XL)
Nonselective (Beta 1 and Beta 2
receptors):
carteolol (Cartrol)
carvedilol (Coreg)
labetalol (Normodyne)
nadolol (Corgard)
penbutolol (Levotol)
pindolol (Visken)
propranolol (Inderal)
sotalol (Betapace)
timolol (Blocadren)
Beta₂ Adrenergic Agonists .. 110, 111
Nonselective Adrenergic:
epinephrine (Adrenalin)
Nonselective Beta₂ Adrenergic:
isoproterenol (Isuprel)
Selective B₂:
albuterol (Proventil, Ventolin)
bitolterol (Tornalate)
isoetharine (Bronkosol)
metaproterenol (Alupent)

pirbuterol (Maxair)
salmeterol (Severent)
terbutaline (Brethine, Bricanyl)
Beta Blockers (Undesirable Effects)..... *59*
Beta Blocker Actions 58
Bile Acid Sequestrants 94, 95
cholestyramine (Questran)
colestipol (Colestid)
Biologic Response Modifiers 174, 175
interferon-alfa (Roferon-A, Alferon N)
interferon-beta (Betaseron),
interferon-gamma (Actimmune)
Bronchodilators .... See *drug specific*
category
Bulk Forming Agent 208, *209*
psyllium (Metamucil)

C

Calcium 316, *317*
calcium carbonate (Caltrate, Chooz,
Equilet, OsCAl, Oystercal, Tums)
Calcium Channel Blockers 60, *61*
amlodipine (Norvasc)
bepridil (Vascor)
diltiazem (Cardizem)
felodipine (Plendil)
isradipine (DynaCirc)
nicardipine (Cardene)
nifedipine (Procardia)
nimodipine (Nimotop)
nisoldipine (Sular)
verapamil (Isoptin, Calan)
Cardiac Glycoside 26, 27
digitoxin (Crystodigin)
digoxin (Lanoxin)
Cardiovascular Agents 25–75
Central Alpha₂ Agonists 62, 63
clonidine (Catapres)
guanabenz (Wytensin)
guanfacine (Tenex)

phytonadione (AquaMEPHYTON)
potassium acetate (Potassium acetate)
potassium chloride (Kaochlor, K-Dur,
    K-Lor, Klotrix, K-Lyte/Cl, Slow-K)
potassium gluconate (Kaon)
pyridoxine (vitamin B_6)

X

aminophylline (theophylline,
    ethylenediamine)
theophylline Immediate Release:
Aerolate
Slo-Phyllin
Theolair
Extended Release:
Slo-Bid
Theo-Dur
Theo-24
Uni-Dur
Uniphyl

PHARMACEUTICAL INDEX

Feeling ANXIOUS About Learning Pharmacology?

A mount to remember is too much

N CLEX-RN® —Ready for the pharmacology changes?

X ero information is being remembered

I don't even know where to begin!

O verwhelmed

U nsure of yourself

S cared

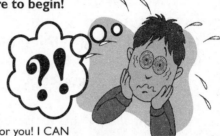

If your answer is YES, this program is for you! I CAN Publishing, Inc. can now bring to your school, nursing organization, or hospital the popular and most sought after 1 day program, **Pharmacology Made Insanely Easy**. We developed this program to make learning pharmacology fun, easy, and memorable. We want you to relax and laugh even while you are studying a challenging topic. Since the NCLEX-RN® has increased the percentage of questions evaluating pharmacology, we want to provide you with a program to increase your confidence in answering questions successfully as well as to enhance clinical practice.

What are participants saying about the program?

"Wow! I finally understand pharmacokinetics and it was actually fun to learn!"

"This program saved me on the NCLEX-RN®! I was able to remember to prioritize my drugs."

"I will never forget cephalosporins thanks to "CEF/CEPH the GIANT"!

"I was always nervous about drug-drug interactions, but I am leaving this program with much more confidence."

"This has been the most interactive course I have ever experienced. Where were you when I was struggling to stay awake while reading my pharmacology text books?"

How Do I Register?

Call **866.428.5589** and register now. For additional information visit our web page at **www.icanpublishing.com**. Coordinate a program at your school for 40 or more participants and receive a **FREE** course. Members of the Student Nurses' Association will receive a discount.

I CAN Publishing, Inc.
P. O. Box 6192 • Bossier City, LA 71171 • 866.428.5589
www.icanpublishing.com

People learn in many different ways.
We want to tell you about our books because our business is to help you PASS.
www.icanpublishing.com

NURSING MADE INSANELY EASY, 4th Ed. is a pocket-sized book, chock full of drawings and information streamlining nursing and allied health education with an EASY totally different bottom line approach to concepts.

E   essential concepts assist learners to prepare for exams, exit exams, and NCLEX®.

A   assist nursing graduates to remember health and disease concepts.

S   special images per page with essential concepts on the opposite page.

Y   your learning is memorable and fun.

Turn the page for a sneak preview from *Nursing Made Insanely Easy*, 4th Edition. We hope you enjoy these few snapshots from our book. As you will be able to see from these pages, learning difficult nursing concepts can truly be made fun and insanely easy!

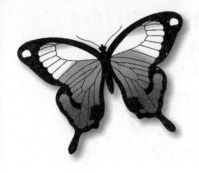

M any of life's failures are people who did not realize how close they were to success when they gave up.

Unknown

PRIORITIZING

We want to introduce you to "MERRY MANAGER". She will be the nurse manager that will accompany you on your journey through out these first two chapters. As you can see by looking at her, she is positive both in her management style as well as in her thinking. She is outcome oriented and always attempts to understand the concerns of her nursing staff. "MERRY" is indeed one of those eagles that every nurse wants to emulate. Join us as we begin our journey through this "INSANELY EASY" and FUN book. Thank you for selecting this book for your journey! Let's get started with prioritizing nursing care.

Nurses must be able to make decisions regarding how to prioritize nursing care. Nurses are daily faced with the challenge regarding which client should be assessed (**FIRST**).

F *FIND HYPOXIA*–When the nurse has several clients to provide care for, oxygenation is always an immediate concern. Hypoxia may be a result of cardiac or respiratory complications. Physiological changes such as vital signs, skin color, or capillary refill are a few of the assessments the nurse would anticipate. Another assessment the nurse may anticipate may be an increase in anxiety or confusion. When there was no alteration in sensorium prior to the current medical condition, this clinical change may strongly represent hypoxia!

I *IMMUNOCOMPROMISED*–If there are 4 clients, none of which are hypoxic, but one client is receiving chemotherapy or is immunocompromised from another medication or medical condition, then this client should be evaluated first. The objective is to prevent infections from being transferred to the client.

R *REAL BLEEDING*–A client that is hemorrhaging from a trauma, surgery, etc. is also a priority. This client will present with changes in the vital signs, skin color, temperature, urine output, etc. which will result in alteration in tissue and organ perfusion. BLEEDING is BAD for the client! Let's get on with the care!

S *SAFETY*–Any client who is at risk for injury from increased intracranial pressure or confusion from delirium or dementia would be important to assess first. A toddler playing with a balloon would also be at risk for injury.

T *TRY INFECTION*–If a client is septic with a high fever, and has an order for blood cultures and antibiotics, this client may be the priority to assess first. The priority for this client is to obtain blood cultures as ordered prior to starting the antibiotic therapy.

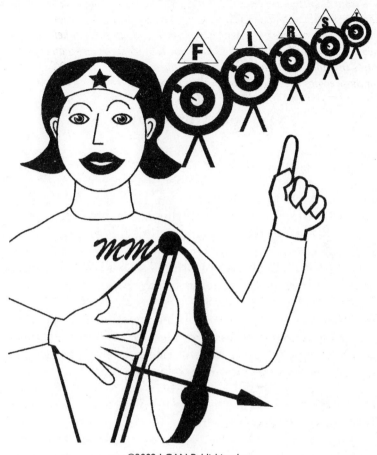

©2002 I CAN Publishing, Inc.

MERRY MANAGER is our STAR manager, because she has the qualities that we believe are so important in any manager.

S **STRENGTH** to grow, help and allow others to grow
T **THE "HAPPINESS FACTOR"** (comfortable in her own shoes, is not a victim and does not blame)
A **A VISIONARY** that can think "out of the box"
R **REACTIVE LAST**, proactive first

DISASTER PLAN

A disaster plan needs to be activated when there is a life threatening risk and a large number of clients must be evacuated from the hospital, assisted living units, etc. "MERRY" needs a way to remember which clients to remove first from the rooms. **ABC** will assist in organizing this information!

A *AMBULATORY*–The priority is to evacuate the largest volume of clients initially.

B *BED RIDDEN*–The bed ridden clients will be the next group to be evacuated from the rooms. Actually, the ambulatory group may be able to assist in getting this group evacuated more quickly.

C *CRITICAL CARE*–The last group of clients to be evacuated will be the critically ill.

The ultimate objective in a disaster plan is to evacuate volumes of clients. If the clients with numerous tubes and IVs are evacuated initially, this will slow the process down. Fewer clients will be safely rescued from the disaster.

DISASTER PLAN

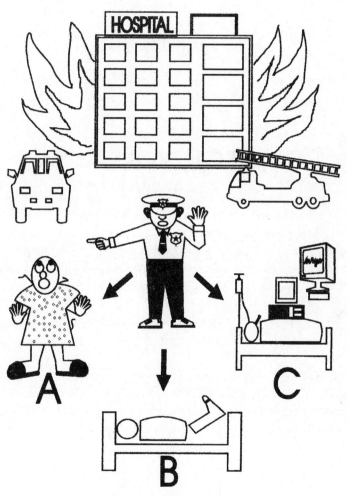

©2002 I CAN Publishing, Inc.

CRUTCH WALKING

Remembering how to instruct the client to use crutches while walking up and down the stairs is "INSANELY EASY". Just look at our friend, Charlie, with his crutches on the next page. He is putting his good leg up on the stair first "UP TO HEAVEN"! When he goes down, his bad leg will go first! Remember, "BAD GOES TO YOU KNOW WHERE".